FRUIT
INFUSED
WATER

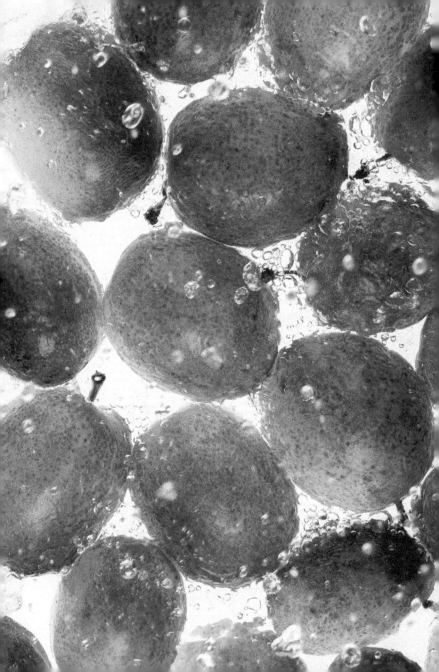

FRUIT INFUSED WATER

98 DELICIOUS RECIPES FOR YOUR FRUIT INFUSER WATER PITCHER

Susan Marque

ROCKRIDGE PRESS

Photo credits: Michael van Emde Boas/Stockfood, pg. 2; Rhonda Adkins/Stocksy, pg. 6; Nadine Greef/Stocksy, pg. 11; Shutterstock, pg. 16; Shutterstock pg. 21; Pavel Gramatikov/Stocksy, pg. 22; Shutterstock, pg. 31; Pavel Gramatikov/Stocksy, pg. 34; Shutterstock, pg. 40; Shutterstock, pg. 46 (left); B & J/Stocksy, pg. 46–47 (center); Davide Illini/Stocksy, pg. 60 (left); Shutterstock, pg. 60–61 (center); Hilde Mèche/Stockfood, pg. 74 (left); Nataša Mandić/Stocksy, pg. 74–75 (center); Shutterstock, pg. 88 (left); Jeff Wasserman/Stocksy, pg. 88–89 (center); Shutterstock, pg. 102 (left); Maya Visnyei/Stockfood, pg. 102–103 (center); Ina Peters/Stocksy, pg. 116 (left); Walter Cimbal/Stockfood, pg. 116–117 (center); Shutterstock, pg. 130 (left); Ina Peters/Stocksy, pg. 130–131 (center); Maximilian Stock Ltd/Stockfood, pg. 144 (left); Shutterstock, pg. 144–145 (center); Nataša Mandić/Stocksy, pg. 158 (left); Jeff Wasserman/Stocksy, pg. 158–159 (center); Shutterstock, pg. 172 (left); Reema Desai/Stocksy, pg. 172–173 (center); Kelsey Skiver/Stockfood, pg. 184 (left); Sara Remington/Stocksy, pg. 184–185 (center); Nataša Mandić/Stocksy, pg. 198.

ISBN: Print 978-1-62315-469-1 | eBook 978-1-62315-470-7

For Mom and Dad

Contents

PART TWO: THE RECIPES

HOW TO USE THIS BOOK

Fruit Infused Water was designed to provide you with a quick and easy introduction to fruit-infused water. Within the pages of this book you will learn the basics about what infusing is and what benefits it may have for your body.

On page 23 you will learn which INGREDIENTS are recommended for infusion as well as those that tend not to work.

Page 18 includes recommendations regarding which type of WATER to use for your infusions.

If you want to GET STARTED RIGHT AWAY, you will find simple instructions in chapter 3, "Use Your Infusion," on page 35.

Once you learn how to use your INFUSER, you will be ready to move on to chapter 4, "One-Step Infusions," on page 47.

For more FRUIT INFUSION RECIPES, see chapter 5 through chapter 11.

If you are looking for recommendations about what type of infuser to purchase, check the RESOURCES section on page 200 in the back of this book.

Introduction

Water infusions have probably been around as long as humans, if you consider that water most likely sat inside shells before cups, absorbing a hint of the coconut or gourd. Dropping a lemon slice into your glass before ice water was poured as you sat down in a restaurant was considered elegant, and it was simply practical in countries where lemon could disinfect the water. Eventually spas came to realize how refreshing fruit infusions could be and how happy they made their clients. Now you can make your own infusions at home that just might rival your previous beverage favorites.

Each one of the recipes in this book is a guide to get you started making your own simple and delicious fruit infusions. Feel free to get creative in mixing and matching elements from one recipe to another. After all, it is your taste that matters. Infusions are a great way to get a little extra benefit from your water. They have helped many people enjoy increasing their H_2O intake, and there are reports of improved energy levels, clearer skin, and relief from minor ailments such as headaches and other pains.

Make a game of trying a new fruit or new combination and enjoy gathering new items for your infusions. Take advantage of your local farmers' market and talk with the farmers—often you will find organic farmers whose methods go above and beyond the standards set by the Food and Drug Administration (FDA) for organic farming, but for one reason or another, they have not yet received their certification. Using the freshest and healthiest ingredients is the best way to get the most out of your fruit-infused water. If you are curious about what fruit-infused water tastes like or what health benefits it may provide for you, this book is the perfect place to start. So settle in and start reading to learn how to incorporate fruit-infused water into your dietary routine.

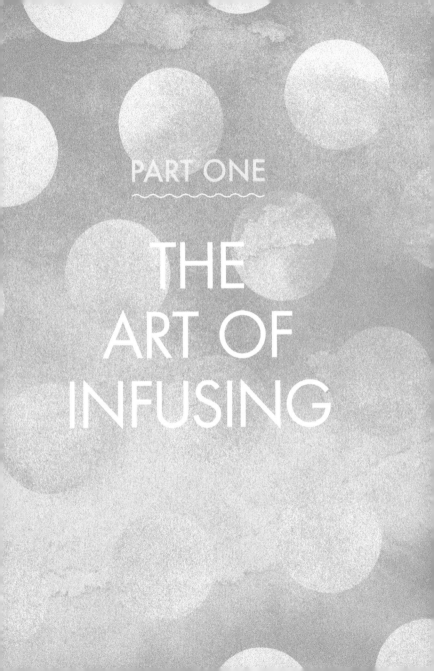

PART ONE

THE
ART OF
INFUSING

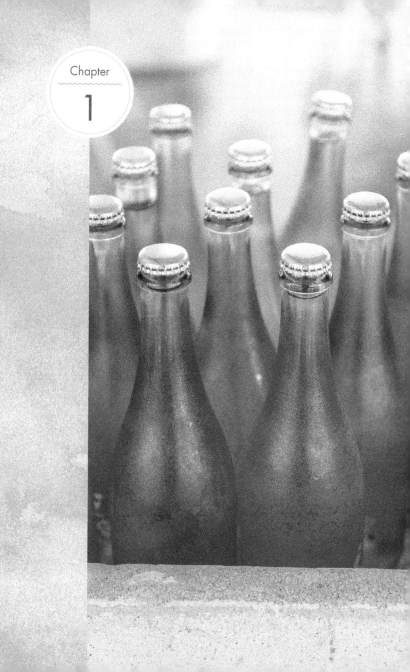

Chapter

1

The Beauty of Water

The Stuff of Life

About 70 percent of the planet we live on is covered by water, and each of our bodies is made up of 60–70 percent H_2O. Staying healthy means staying hydrated. Water is the largest component of almost every part of your body, and while air is slightly more important to sustain life, you will not survive very long without water. You already know that the hotter it gets, the more you sweat, and the more water you need to rehydrate. Sweating is your body's way of cooling down when it gets hot—it eliminates excess heat and helps regulate body temperature.

You might not be aware, however, that water is also needed for proper digestion. It has been said that digestion is the "seat of our health," and without enough water, absorption and elimination will be impaired. It is important to get enough water between meals, before meals, and when exercising to make sure everything in your body keeps running smoothly. Water also helps lubricate the joints and carries nutrients to your cells. It carries waste out of the cells and helps keep you feeling vibrant and looking clear and fresh. Getting enough water is one of the most important actions we can take to keep our bodies in great working order.

Beverages contribute the largest amount of water a person consumes in a day—about 80 percent of your total water intake. Food contributes about 20 percent to total water intake; that number is slightly higher when you eat mostly vegetables, fruits, and whole grains (the kind that are cooked in water) as the basis of your diet. Eating a diet full of processed foods causes your body to need even more water to rehydrate flour particles so they can then be digested and the available nutrients absorbed. Not getting enough water can slow down metabolic functions in the body so that waste and fats are not properly eliminated. This is one reason why people who quench their thirst with soft drinks loaded with sugar and do not drink enough water often struggle with fat elimination.

Water is useful in maintaining an ideal weight. It's easy to confuse hunger and thirst—you may often think you are hungry when you are really thirsty. Drinking adequate amounts of water can help you cut down on the amount of food you consume, which typically leads to a leaner, healthier physique, especially when the overall diet is healthy.

One reason many people cite for not drinking enough water is the fact that it doesn't have much natural flavor. If water doesn't taste good, then it is difficult to drink as much as your body needs. Water acts like a delivery system—putting chemicals and pollution into your body in the form of soft drinks requires your hardworking organs to filter out what the body cannot use. If you truly want to take care of your body, you should only put into it substances that will support its healthy function, not hamper it. When you take care of your body by drinking enough water, you will see more of the results you want, such as clear skin, a flat tummy, great energy, stamina, strength, and more. Water is often overlooked as a nutrient, but it is one of the most important ingredients available.

Better than Soda

From *Sugar Blues* to *Fat Chance*, there are plenty of books depicting the dangers of sugar. Processed white or brown sugar comes in a variety of forms with many different names, but all of them are addictive. Sugar is so addictive, in fact, that scientists have proven that its effect on the body is not very different from that of cocaine and other highly addictive substances. Given this information, you can see how sugar might be a contributing factor to many modern-day ailments. Diabetes, heart disease, metabolic syndrome, and weight gain are all associated with the overconsumption of sugar. Added sugars in the American diet come from many sources: candy makes up only 6.1 percent of those added sugars, while sodas contribute a whopping 35.7 percent. Sugar is even added to already

Hydrate!

You have probably been told that you should drink eight glasses of water per day—this is the standard recommendation for those following the average American diet. It is important to realize, however, that everyone has different water needs. According to the Institute of Medicine, men need up to thirteen 8-ounce servings of water per day while women need only about nine 8-ounce servings (Institute of Medicine, 2004).

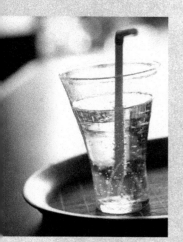

Dehydration is dangerous. You begin to feel fatigued when your body's water supply is depleted by just 1 percent of your body weight. After that, your mental function becomes impaired with only a 2 percent loss of water. If a person loses 10 percent of his body weight in water, he could die.

You know you are probably not drinking enough water if you are experiencing symptoms of dehydration such as a fast heart rate, fatigue, dry skin, dry mouth, or dry eyes. Be sure to increase your water intake by drinking water; eating water-rich foods; and cutting down on consuming dry, hard, and baked items. To make sure you get enough water each day, fill a 3-quart pitcher and keep it in the refrigerator. Refill your glass throughout the day and use the pitcher as a visual guide to see if you are drinking enough.

Note: In cases of illness involving diarrhea, vomiting, high fever, burns, or trauma, the body's need for water will increase significantly. You should also drink more water during prolonged physical activity and when it is very hot outside.

sweet foods like fruit juice and other beverages, making them a burden on the body instead of a good source of fuel.

Water is a substance that allows your body to absorb nutrition and to utilize the nutrients it needs. It helps maintain a clear state of mind so that you can focus and be productive. Sugar-laden drinks have the opposite effect—and they can make you fat. When you consume sugar, your body releases a hormone called insulin that pulls the sugar from your blood so it can be utilized for energy; excess sugar is stored as fat. The more sugar you consume, the higher your insulin levels become, leading to increased fat storage. In addition to increasing fat storage, higher insulin levels also prevent the hormone leptin from doing its job. Leptin is responsible for signaling to the brain that you are full and that you should stop eating. If leptin doesn't get this message to the brain, you will likely continue to ingest the very things that are causing your insulin levels to spike.

The Internet is full of stories of people who quit drinking sugary sodas and lost 10, 15, or even 25 pounds in just a few months. Countless people have found that switching from soda to water helped them release excess weight at the healthy rate of one to two pounds per week. Many of these individuals also experienced a surprising side effect—after just two weeks, water started to taste better than their sugary drinks ever did. The 2014 documentary *Fed Up* created a 10-day challenge to help people completely give up all refined sugar—even including relinquishing smoothies and juice for 10 days. (Fruit-infused water with its tiny fructose content is okay and encouraged.) The creators of the documentary state that you ought to feel better in just one to two days and that the sugar cravings ought to dissipate within three weeks.

When water tastes great it is far easier to drink more of it, stay hydrated, and enjoy the reward of a body that is functioning optimally. One of the great things about infusing water with fruit is that it provides additional nutritional benefits with very little sugar. More importantly, it is far more fun to drink infused water than plain water, so most people find they will drink more of it. With fruit-infused water you can achieve endless variety, and it can be cheaper than supporting your soda habit. If you can wait out the first three weeks of transition, switching to water from any type of sugary beverage will become easy and satisfying. Your tastes will change and the fruit infusions will become sweeter than you thought they were at the beginning of the transition. By using fruit infusions to make your water fun to drink you will find that the health benefits you gain are the sweetest infusion of all.

Many Waters

Purified water is often filtered to remove chlorine, fluoride, and other chemicals that are put into municipal drinking water to make it safe for human consumption. The use of these chemicals was mandated to keep people safe from harmful bacteria and to help prevent dental cavities. Well water is often naturally filtered and typically does not contain any additives. It has a fresh taste and is generally safe to drink from the tap, just like purified water. Putting tap water into the refrigerator for a couple of hours may help dissipate the chlorine, but it won't remove fluoride or other impurities. While these substances are designed to keep you safe, there is some controversy regarding whether they are really good for you.

Use the water that makes you feel great about drinking it. For those who just want to remove chlorine, a simple carbon filter might do the trick. Pur or Brita are two of the most popular brands of water filter, available as a pitcher-style filter or one that mounts to the countertop or under the sink. Just remember to change the filters regularly and always pour out the first two pitchers of water that you put through them, as they can contain some carbon residue. Tap water is generally tested to be safe, and you can request a report from your city if you want to know what is in your water.

Starting with quality ingredients will give you quality results. If you like the taste and feel of filtered water, you may wish to invest in a home filtering system that is more powerful than a carbon filter. You won't be soaking chlorine in through your skin when you shower with this filtration system, and you can fill your water infusion pitcher from any sink in your home. In the end, the choice it up to you—go with what you are most comfortable with.

Make It Bubbly

There is some concern that drinking carbonated water will prevent calcium absorption and lead to bone problems like osteoporosis. Detractors of this theory, however, are quick to point out that the study used to draw this conclusion looked only at carbonated drinks like cola, not carbonated water. Carbonating your water can be a fun alternative to flat water. With fruit infusions it can make drinking your water a treat.

There are several ways to use carbonated water in your infusions. For example, you might purchase a sparkling water such as San Pellegrino, Ty Nant, or Perrier. Or you can purchase a seltzer bottle, like one you may have seen in a 1950s film or at your grandparents' house, to make your own carbonated water. SodaStream is a modern version of the seltzer bottle and offers you control over how much fizz you put into your water. There is even a do-it-yourself method that does not involve forcing carbon dioxide into the water with pressure. Instead, you get the right mix of baking soda and vinegar to do the fizzing. This method can be tricky, however, so you may want to stick with water that is already carbonated to see if you like it before you invest in anything complicated.

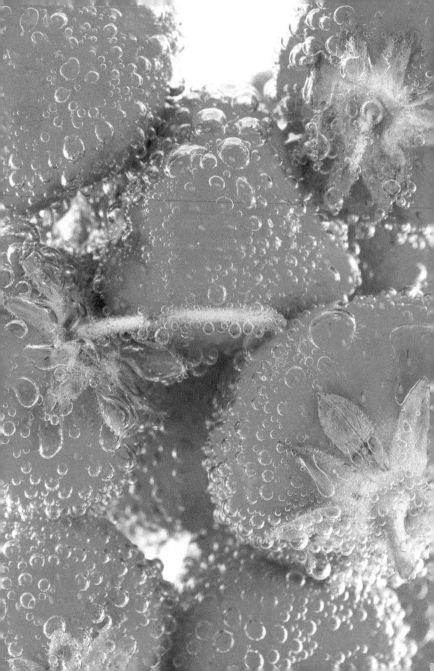

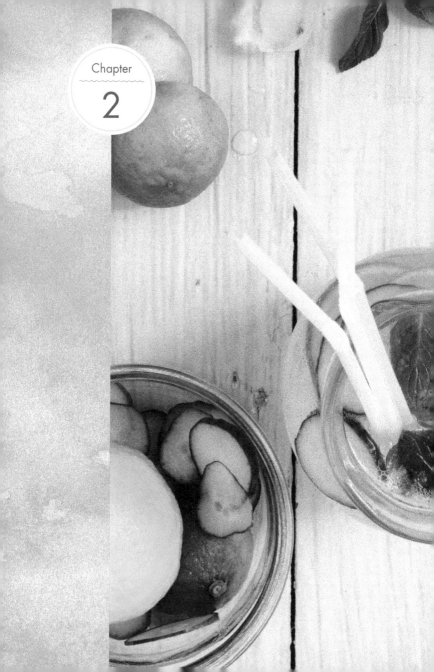

Chapter

2

Natural Flavors

Ingredients & Vitamins

What foods are best for infusion? Unlike tea, infusions do not use heat to draw flavors out of dried ingredients. For fruit-infused beverages, it is often best to use fresh ingredients that are porous and juicy. While you might like to add a little bit of dry cocoa powder, cinnamon, cayenne pepper, or other spice, the main ingredients should be delicate and able to mix with the water without much effort. Melons, citrus fruits, berries, and even bananas are all going to infuse beautifully to give your water a hint of flavor. Once you see how easy and fun these recipes are, you can choose according to your taste, preference, and the benefits of each ingredient.

When making infusions it is best to limit the ingredients to get a distinctive flavor. Too many ingredients all at once can literally muddy the water, but a few ingredients will give you endless refreshment. You might want to experiment with mixing in vegetables with the fruits to see how that tastes. If you think peas mixed with mint and pear sounds appealing, or carrots, lime, and sage—try it.

Citrus fruits are a natural choice for infusion; they have a high juice content that will mix nicely with water in an infusion. Recommended citrus fruits for infusion include:

Grapefruit: Known to help lower blood sugar and support the liver, grapefruit can also aid poor digestion.

Lemon: Supports the liver and aids digestion. Lemon has antiseptic and antimicrobial properties as well as a cooling effect.

Lime: Similar to lemons, with even stronger benefits for the liver. While lemon and lime both contain water-soluble citric acid, they are considered alkalizing for the body.

Orange: High in vitamin C, oranges can help cleanse the liver and blood.

Tangerine/Mandarin: Some say mandarins are good for curing hiccups. They are definitely good for the liver and digestion, as are other citrus fruits. Mandarins are also good for quenching thirst and clearing chest congestion.

Melons are so full of water that they are easily muddled and infused. Recommended melons for infusion include:

Cantaloupe: Rich in potassium, cantaloupes are cooling and, like all melons, can lift depression. They have diuretic properties and also contain adenosine, an anticoagulant.

Crenshaw, Casaba, Honeydew: All have similar health benefits to cantaloupe.

Cucumber: Diuretic and cooling, cucumber helps purify the blood. Contains erepsin, a digestive enzyme that breaks down protein into its amino acids.

Watermelon: Relieves thirst and lifts depression. Watermelon is a good source of vitamins A and C and potassium.

Berries, with their delicate nature, are perfect for water infusions. They have high water content and intense flavors that mix easily with a little muddling. Recommended berries for infusion include:

Blackberries: Known to increase cognitive function, blackberries are rich in vitamin C. They are astringent and mildly diuretic.

Blueberries: Good source of vitamins A and C and manganese. Blueberries have bacteria-fighting capabilities similar to cranberries that can be good for urinary tract infections.

Raspberries: Strengthen the kidneys, cleanse the blood, and benefit the liver. Raspberries are touted as being able to strengthen vision.

Strawberries: Have both antiviral and tranquilizing effects. Strawberry scents are often used in dentistry to calm the nerves, and the extract may be rubbed onto the teeth and gums to remove tartar and strengthen teeth.

Any fruits that you enjoy can be good for infusions. Softer fruits are easier to muddle and thus impart more of their essence to your drink. Other fruits recommended for infusion include:

Apple: Cleansing to the liver, apples are cooling and good for digestion. Apples are good for relieving thirst and can reduce a fever.

Apricot: A good source of vitamin A and carotene. Apricots can be used to ease a dry throat or dry cough.

Banana: Can ease thirst and treat constipation. Bananas are high in potassium.

Cherry: Contains iron, phosphorus, potassium, calcium, and vitamin A. Cherries are astringent and are a warming food said to increase energy.

Chile: These vegetables are cooling and can improve the appetite. They are rich in antioxidants, vitamins A and C, and also lycopene, which may help fight certain types of cancer.

Coconut: Along with wonderful fatty acids, coconut contains manganese, copper, and potassium. Antifungal and antibacterial, coconut provides energy and is rich in antioxidants.

Cranberry: High in antioxidants, cranberries are a good source of proanthocyanidins that inhibit bacteria from adhering to the urinary tract or bladder.

Fig: Aids in digestion and can treat constipation. High in potassium, figs have been used to treat boils and hemorrhoids.

Grape: Benefits the kidneys, liver, and bones. Grapes are easily digested and contain vitamins A, C, and B-complex.

Kiwi: Can relieve thirst and cool the body. Kiwis are very high in vitamin C and also contain magnesium and potassium. They are high in antioxidants and can lower your risk for blood clots.

Mango: A good source of vitamins A and C and potassium. Mangoes are cooling and can quench thirst.

Nectarine: High in vitamins A and C. Nectarines are a good source of antioxidants and can be sweeter than peaches.

Papaya: Contains carpaine, a compound thought to have anti-tumor activity. Like cherries, papayas are a warming, rather than cooling, fruit. High in papain, an enzyme that helps break down proteins and aids digestion.

Peach: High in vitamins A and C as well as calcium. Peaches are astringent and are touted to tighten tissues.

Pear: Pectin in pears can reduce cholesterol and flush out toxins. Pears are excellent for digestion and alleviating constipation or fluid retention.

Persimmon: Good source of potassium and vitamin A. Persimmon can relieve a dry hacking cough, help moisten the body, and help curb certain types of bleeding, such as a bleeding hemorrhoid.

Pineapple: Contains the anti-inflammatory enzyme bromelain. Aided by the high proportion of manganese found in pineapple, bromelain is known to help digest starches or proteins and also can soothe a sore throat.

Plum: Aids digestion and relieves thirst. Plums are helpful for liver problems and can increase iron absorption.

Pomegranate: High in potassium. The pomegranate can foster the production of red blood cells, strengthen the bladder, and sooth mouth ulcers.

Fresh herbs also make a flavorful addition to your infusions. Herbs offer flavor along with many wonderful benefits. Recommended herbs for infusion include:

Basil: Rich in antioxidants, this herb can reduce swelling and treat mild depression. Basil can also be used to calm the nerves, aid digestion, and even ward off bacterial infections.

Lavender: Calming for both mind and body. Lavender can be used to ease anxiety, depression, exhaustion, irritability, and headaches. It also is good for digestion and can lower fevers.

Mint: Known as a digestive aid, mint can also disperse pathogens and cool the body as well as helping clear nasal passages.

Parsley: Known for freshening breath, parsley is high in vitamins A and C and very high in iron. It can strengthen the teeth and purify the blood.

Rosemary: Supports mental function and memory. May also help ease muscle pain, sore throat, cough, and heartburn.

Sage: A decongestant with antimicrobial properties. Sage can be used to reduce menopausal symptoms, especially hot flashes. It is also used to calm the nerves.

Thyme: Commonly used for coughs, sore throats, and indigestion. Thyme is thought to calm the mind and even ease arthritis.

Other ingredients you will find in these recipes are added for flavor and taste as well as their health benefits. Some of the additional ingredients you will find in recipes include:

Cinnamon: Can lower blood sugar and increase vitality. While it is not recommended for pregnant women to consume too much cinnamon, it is good for clearing intestinal gas, can help fight fungal infections, and may help prevent Alzheimer's disease.

Cocoa: Rich in phenols, it can lower blood pressure, help clear arterial plaque, and trigger good feelings.

Ginger: Like mint, ginger is known for stimulating and aiding digestion while also being good for circulation and respiration. It can help alleviate motion sickness and nausea, reduce blood pressure, and is even used as a treatment for a cold or fever.

Vanilla: Can be used to treat fever and intestinal gas as well as being an aphrodisiac. Vanilla's fragrant aroma is soothing and may help boost self-confidence.

In Season

Depending on where you live, summer can be the most bountiful time of year for fruits. Melons, berries, stone fruits, and citrus are usually easy to find in stores and farmers' markets. As fall descends, you will be able to find fresh berries, and you can pick apples, pears, cranberries, persimmons, and pomegranates. During the cold winter months, warmer places provide lovely citrus, dates, and bananas, and when spring arrives, so do the strawberries, melons, apricots, and mangoes.

Going Organic

While there is no definitive scientific evidence stating that organics are significantly higher in nutrients than their conventional counterparts, even experts agree that organic tastes superior. There is consistently richer flavor in organic produce. If you ask organic farmers, they will say that the great taste comes from the care they give the soil—the plants absorb the extra nutrients in the soil and they are passed on to you. According to a

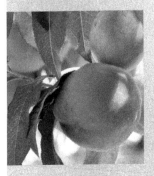 study led by Professor Carlo Leifert of Newcastle University, organic fruits and vegetables contain as much as 40 percent more antioxidants than conventional produce (Weil, 2014). Antioxidants are powerful molecules that protect your cells from free-radical damage and may also help increase your resistance to disease and aging.

You are not consuming pesticides, sprays, or genetically modified organisms when you choose to eat organic. By eating clean produce you can rest assured that it was grown without doing harm to the environment, and that feels pretty good, too.

To pick the best fruits, and make the tastiest water infusions, you need to watch out for a few things.

Color. Fruits are colorful. They come in a huge variety of hues, from reds and oranges to blues and greens. You can often tell what berries will be the sweetest, what stone fruits will be more sugary than sour, and even which kiwi will taste the best, just by their outside appearance. A dark, rich-looking fruit is usually what you want to find: the apricot that looks more orange than yellow, the fully red strawberries that have grown enough to develop a sweet taste. Even a kiwi that is sweet will look a little darker than the sour, slightly lighter ones.

Firmness. Think of fruits like people. Youth is thought to be vibrant because our skin is soft, firm, and radiant. Fruits that are ripe will have that youthful glow as well. With stone fruits, the skins are often taught but yield to the touch. Apples are shiny and very firm. When stored properly, apples will stay crisp. Leave the ones that feel soft to the touch. When picking a pineapple, you want to be able to pluck out a top leaf fairly easily. If you can't pluck a leaf, it is most likely going to be sour.

Sound. Knock on a melon and you should hear a hollow sound (not the knocking sound of hitting your knuckles against wood). Ask your grocer if you can't tell the difference, because there is nothing quite like the wonderful sweet taste of a good melon.

Don't Toss That Fruit!

Don't want to toss out your ingredients after making a batch of fruit-infused water? You can reuse the same ingredients and add more water as you drink it down, then let it sit a bit longer to infuse again. After a full day or two, however, you will want to begin with fresh ingredients. To replenish the flavor that becomes diluted from repeated use, add a bit more of the fresh ingredients to the mixture, muddling when appropriate. If you are using lemon as one of your components, you may be able to reuse your mixture for up to a third or even a fourth day, since lemon can keep the other ingredients from spoiling.

A Little Something Sweet

For added sweetness you may wish to use stevia, or perhaps agave, honey, brown rice syrup, or maple sugar. While there are mixed reviews of artificial sweeteners, it is best to steer clear of anything claiming to be natural that sounds like a chemical. Stevia is the one sweetener that will not contribute known carcinogens or any artificial ingredients, even though it has zero calories, contains no sugar, and is very sweet. If you use a bit of honey, maple syrup, brown rice syrup, coconut sugar, or agave, you might want to give your infusion a stir before serving, since it takes a little more effort to get the thicker sweeteners fully incorporated.

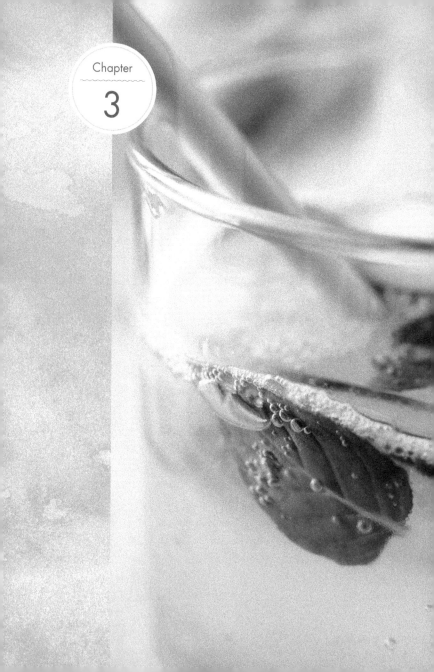

Chapter

3

Use Your Infusion

The Fruit Infusion Pitcher

Of course you can make fruit-infused water without an infusion pitcher, but with so many to choose from at a reasonable price, having an infusion pitcher is a sound investment. It is a great tool to make your infusions taste wonderful while also giving you the ease of filtering and quick cleaning. You won't need a strainer when you have this type of pitcher, and if you get one of the portable models, you can also drink out of it. In the long run it saves you time and effort, making the infusion process much easier. Plus, you can use your infusion pitcher in unique ways to create a variety of delicious beverages. For example, you can make infused iced tea or lemonade in addition to your water infusions.

Most infusion pitchers have a core container or a container at the bottom where you put your ingredients. The holes should be small enough that seeds or leaves will not float out into your water but the essence of the fruits and herbs will—if there is a filter, it should be covered with mesh. Portable infusers are easily shaken and there is usually no need for muddling, since the fruit will be compressed when you immerse the ingredient container into the main water body. Portable infusers are great for those who want infused water on the go. You can refill your infuser and reuse the fruit, then toss it out with one quick motion and start fresh later or the next day.

A few brands of infusers come with a muddler. This handy tool allows you to crush your ingredients to release additional flavor—more flavor than you would get by simply slicing and adding your ingredients to the mix. For those who want strong-tasting recipes, muddling is the way to go. For others who want to reuse ingredients for several days, you can infuse the recipe as is, and then muddle on subsequent days to push more flavor into your water. If you don't have an actual muddler, a wooden spoon will work—just not as well, since a muddler has a greater surface area to push directly down the core container of your pitcher.

Some infusion pitchers come with another core that you can keep in the freezer and use to chill your beverages when your pitcher sits on a counter or desk. This is handy when you have company or want to leave your pitcher out all day. Say you are homeschooling your kids and want to be sure they drink plenty of water, or you have a pitcher in your office and find that you drink significantly more liquid when it is cold—one of these cores that you can freeze every night between infusions is a great addition to your pitcher.

10 Tips for a Successful Water Infusion

1. Plan ahead. Buy some extra fruits and fresh herbs every time you go to the grocery store. Put extra fruit on your list so that you have a couple of options.

2. Stock up. Keep a few frozen favorites for when you run out of fresh ingredients. If you grow your own fruits, be sure to freeze your extra harvest instead of giving it away.

3. Remember the rule of three. Up to three ingredients make great-tasting infusions, but too many ingredients can create a muddy, unpleasant taste.

4. Be flexible. If infused water is helping you hydrate and feel great, don't be caught up in doing it perfectly. Some days you might run out of a certain ingredient. Instead of abandoning your infusion, just create your recipe using what you have available. You might surprise yourself with your ingenuity.

5. Infuse overnight. Longer infusions have richer flavors. The easiest way to get an 8- to 12-hour infusion is to set up your pitcher at night so it is all ready in the morning.

6. Create a habit. Remember, it takes 21 to 30 days to create a new habit. You might be replacing your old soda habit with infused water, so a big key to success is staying consistent for 30 days. Set a reminder on your smartphone or set up a system where you remember to get your pitcher ready each day. It's best if you do it at the same time and in the same spot so that you will be more likely to remember to do it.

7. Buy organic. Give your body what it needs and avoid what it doesn't. The few extra pennies that you spend on organic produce pay off with giant dividends over time. If you don't take care of your health now, you may end up with increased medical costs later. If your body has to process out pesticides or genetically modified ingredients, you might not get the benefits of eating healthier. Start with quality foods to create a quality life.

8. Open your mind to new tastes. Often change is met with resistance, but if you push past it, you may find that you like the difference. Lavender vanilla water might appeal to some people instantly, but if you are used to drinking 10 cups of coffee or 10 sodas a day, then it might make you cringe until your palate adjusts. Give the exotic ingredients a go when you have acclimated to daily infused water.

9. Clean your pitcher. While this might seem obvious, many people keep reusing ingredients, tossing out the old and using their pitcher again right away. It's best to give it a good wash between batches, so you don't mix in old flavors or bits of fruit that might be going bad.

10. Keep experimenting. There is a great deal of potential in trying new things, so why do so many people get stuck in ruts? Ruts are safe. Routine is comfortable. The unknown can be scary, but you should keep playing with your infusions to get the most out of them.

Ingredient Prep

Preparing your ingredients for infusions is very simple. Most berries are prewashed—you can just toss them in. With berries such as strawberries, you might want to chop off the green leaves, since they will not be sweet like the berries themselves. The biggest thing to watch out for is dirt—infusions are not fun to drink if there is gritty sand or dirt in your water. If you procured your produce from the farmers' market or from your own garden, just give it a quick rinse to ensure that your beverages will be dirt-free. Rinse all of the berries or herbs in a container at once, and then pat dry the amount you are saving and storing in the refrigerator.

Since you will strain your infusions either by putting the ingredients in the strainer compartment of your infusion pitcher or by using a strainer when you pour from the container into your glass, you may not need to core apples, pears, or other fruits that have cores. To cut a stone fruit such as a peach into neat slices, you need to cut the fruit in half and remove the pit before slicing.

You can cut your infusion ingredients in any way that pleases you as long as they fit easily into your infusion pitcher's core or basket. Thicker slices or chunks will work

Fresh or Frozen?

Is fresh always best? Probably, but frozen isn't bad either. Depending where you live and how you obtain your produce, frozen might be just as viable an option as fresh ingredients. It is important to realize that berries and fruits shipped from California to other parts of the United States are often picked before they are ripe, so they don't bruise and spoil before they reach their destination. If you purchase imported fruits, you may 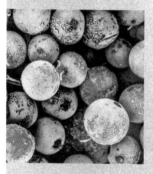 need to give them time to ripen. Fruits that are allowed to ripen on the vine will offer the highest nutritional impact. Many frozen fruits are picked when ripe and then frozen because the freezing process ensures that shipping won't damage the product. No matter how things are shipped, you end up with a lower nutritional content than you would if you could pick your own fruit and take it home. For infusions it is often more about taste than nutrition, however, and you will get great flavors with both fresh and frozen fruits, so find out what you prefer by experimenting.

better if you plan to reuse the ingredients multiple times; thinner slices often impart more of their flavor on the first use. There is no right or wrong when it comes to infusing—it is all up to your personal style and enjoyment.

Handy Equipment

1. Pitcher. Infusions are so simple to make that you can make them in virtually any container you have on hand. A glass pitcher is optimal for both its beauty and functionality. With glass you do not have to worry that any plastic compounds might leach into your beverages. Most water infusion pitchers are made to prevent that from happening, though, even if they do not happen to be glass. A pitcher is easier to pour from than a jar, and while lidded jars can be good for infusions because you can shake them, the lids don't always have a tight seal. Pitchers are a great way to go.

2. Sieve or strainer. This item of equipment ought to be in every kitchen. Many people, hearing the word *strainer*, think of a salad strainer or pasta strainer with large holes for the water to drain through—that is, a colander. A fine mesh strainer or sieve is useful for countless kitchen tasks such as sifting flour to make a light batter, or in the case of infusions, straining out all of the tiny bits that you do not want to drink. Your kitchen would not be complete without an all-purpose strainer or sieve.

3. Muddler. This tool is often shaped like a dowel or a pestle, and it works similarly to a pestle. A muddler is used to mash or break open ingredients to release their flavors. This is a perfect tool for infusions because you want to release the flavor and infuse it in the water.

Serving Suggestions

A beautiful presentation makes anything taste better. Present your water infusions in the best light by using glass pitchers. Clear glass is the safest as it won't leach any chemical residue into your healthy water. Colored glass or glass containers with silicone sleeves or spouts are good, too.

Show off your beautiful infusions by letting them sit out on a table or in the office. The colorful fruit looks beautiful even when you add ice to keep it cool, so be sure to leave the fruits and other items in the water. Another fun way to serve your water infusions is to fill an ice cube tray a little less than all the way full. Add a slice of fruit or a few small berries to each compartment, and then freeze. Then serve your water in glasses with these fruity ice cubes for a colorful, suspended appearance.

Chilled glasses are a fun way to serve your infusions. Add a slice of fruit to each glass, either on the rim or floating. If you are serving a sparkling infusion, adding a straw to the glass can make your presentation feel extra special.

Don't skimp when you are infusing water for yourself. Giving yourself a nice presentation is going to make you feel good, even when no one is watching.

On the Go

Infused water can be strained and poured into any portable water bottle that you have on hand. You can even make infused water directly in a water bottle, but only the specially designed infusion water bottles will have an internal filter to ensure smooth debris-free sipping. Some on-the-go water infusion bottles even come with their own straws, which is great—the more fun your infusion is to drink, the more you will enjoy it and the more hydrated you will become. Be sure to keep your water bottle clean between uses so that you always have the freshest taste possible for your infusions.

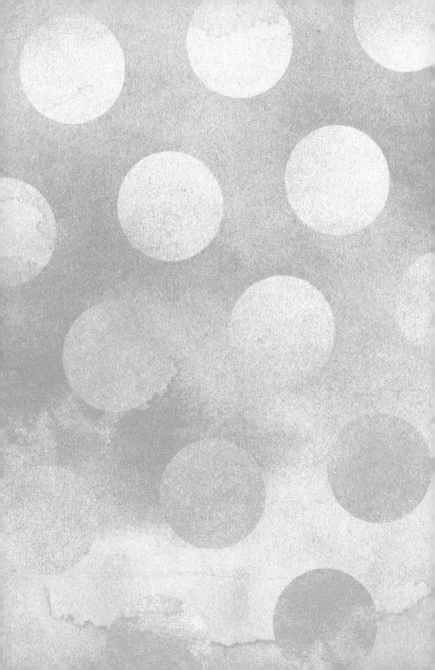

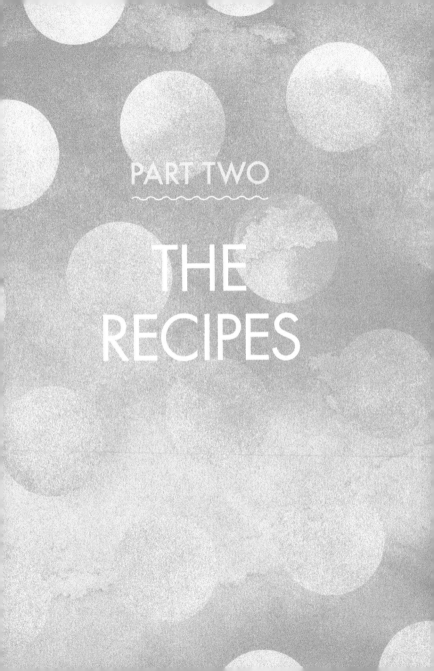

PART TWO

THE
RECIPES

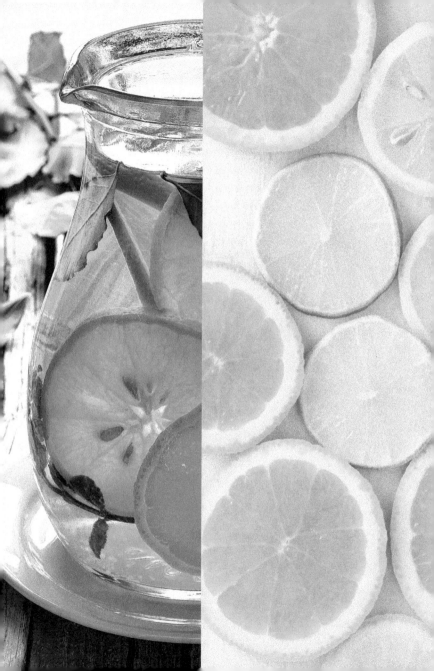

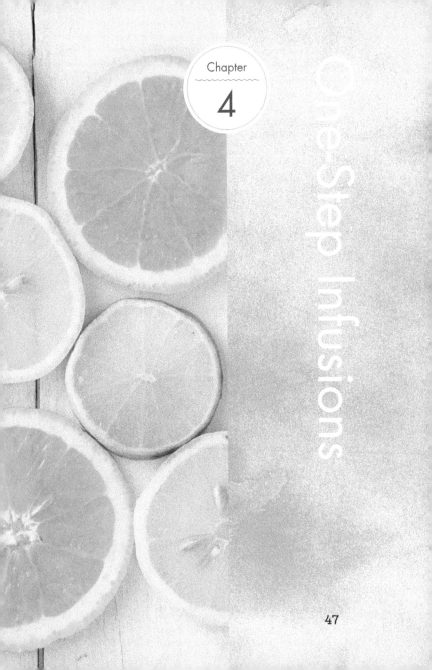

Chapter

4

One-Step Infusions

Water infused with just one fruit or herb is an easy way to start making your own infusions. It is also fun to try a different flavor each day. If you work in an office or go to school, take your on-the-go infuser with you and you will soon start to see others becoming curious about your special water. Taking your infused water with you is a great way to enjoy a refreshing beverage all day long, and it gives you the opportunity to share your newfound joy with others.

As is true with any infusion, the ingredients you choose for a one-step infusion are just as important as the steps you take in preparing them. Muddling (mashing the fruits with a muddler or wooden spoon) is not always necessary, but it may yield a more pronounced flavor. While fresh ingredients are best, it is great to keep a variety of organic frozen fruits in the freezer for the days you run out of ripe produce or when you don't have time to get to the market. Frozen fruits will work better than dried fruits for infusions, but be creative and use what you have on hand to create fun infusions with fresh ingredients.

Orange Water

There is nothing quite as refreshing and sweet as a juicy orange. Filled with sunny vitamin C, orange-infused water can keep a smile on your lips and hydration in your cells. Orange water is beautiful to look at and satisfying to enjoy.

2 or 3 large oranges
8 cups water

Slice the oranges and put the slices in a pitcher.

Cover with water and chill for 2 to 12 hours before serving.

Fruit Infused Water

This is one infusion where you can add more water as you drink it, so you can keep using your orange slices for several days.

Pineapple Water

Makes 8 cups (64 ounces)   Prep time: 1–4 minutes

Great for your digestion, this fun-to-sip water is terrific before, during, and after exercise—you can also use it to energize yourself before a big meeting. Fresh pineapple adds a sweet and refreshing twist to ordinary water that can perk you right up.

2 cups fresh pineapple, chopped
8 cups water

Put the chopped pineapple in a pitcher.

Gently crush the pineapple with a muddler or wooden spoon.

Cover with water and chill for 2 to 12 hours before serving.

One-Step Infusions

Cucumber Water

Makes 8 cups (64 ounces)   Prep time: 5 minutes

Even those who are not too crazy about eating raw cucumber as a snack find that cucumber-infused water is a lovely beverage. It adds just a hint of flavor that makes the water go down smooth and cool.

3 cucumbers, sliced
6 cups ice cubes
2 cups water

Put the cucumber slices in a pitcher.

Put the ice on top of the cucumber to weigh it down.

Pour in the water and chill for 2 to 12 hours
before serving.

There is a trick to having your cucumbers taste sweeter. Cut off about an inch of the vegetable at the stem end, and, holding the cut parts together, briskly rub the two pieces together in a circular motion. White foam will appear around the edges—this foam is a sign that you are drawing out any bitterness from the cucumber.

Blackberry Water

Sweet and tart at the same time, blackberries are terrific when infused in water. Since blackberries are touted as good for the brain, Blackberry Water is the perfect beverage to psych you up for a big meeting—or you can imagine yourself sipping a tall glass while lounging on a sailboat like a superstar. Blackberry Water is great with either still or sparkling water for a refreshing and sugar-free alternative to even the healthiest of sodas.

2 cups fresh blackberries
8 cups water

Put the berries in a pitcher.

Crush the berries slightly with a muddler or wooden spoon.

Pour in the water and chill for 1 to 12 hours before serving.

One-Step Infusions

Mint Water

There are many different types of mint, though the most common type found in US grocery stores is spearmint. Farmers' markets often carry a true peppermint and sometimes even a chocolate mint from Switzerland that is true to its name. Banana mint, lavender mint, and apple mint are exceptional finds as well. If you want to grow your own mint at home, you can order seeds online or find them at your local home and garden supply store.

5 fresh mint sprigs
6 cups ice cubes
2 cups water

Crush the mint leaves with your fingers and put the sprigs in a 10-cup (80-ounce) pitcher.

Put the ice on top of the mint, then pour in the water.

Chill for 1 to 12 hours before serving.

If you have a mint you especially enjoy, put a sprig in a glass of water. It will sprout roots and keep growing, so you can plant it and continue to enjoy your favorite mint.

Fruit Infused Water

Cantaloupe Water

Makes 8 cups (64 ounces)   Prep time: 3 minutes

If you love a sweet melon, cantaloupe water might be your favorite elixir. While the flavor of cantaloupe combines nicely with other ingredients, the simplicity of the single fruit in this infusion is elegant enough for a dinner party and homey in a way that makes it lovely to sip any time of day.

½ ripe cantaloupe, peeled and cubed
8 cups water

Put the cubed cantaloupe into a pitcher.

Muddle the fruit by crushing it slightly with a wooden spoon.

Pour in the water and chill for 1 to 12 hours before serving.

One-Step Infusions

Lemon Water

Makes 8 cups (64 ounces)   Prep time: 3 minutes

Lemon water might seem common, but letting the slices infuse for a few hours creates a richer taste than just a tiny slice floating in a water glass. Sipping on lemon-infused water can curb your appetite and give your whole body the alkalizing benefits of lemon.

3 lemons
8 cups water

Slice the lemons and put them in a pitcher.

Muddle the lemon slices by pressing them with a wooden spoon.

Pour in the water and chill for 1 to 12 hours before serving.

Coconut-Infused Water

Not to be confused with coconut water—the juice of a coconut taken from a palm tree—here you are creating water that is infused with the essence of coconut. If you love coconut, you might even try this with dried pieces of coconut meat, though fresh coconut will give you a brighter taste, which is most likely the type of coconut flavor you are looking for.

> Meat from ½ fresh coconut, chopped
> 8 cups water

Put the coconut meat in a pitcher.

Pour in the water and chill for 3 to 12 hours before serving.

One-Step Infusions

Since coconut is solidly structured, you may wish to eat the coconut chunks even after they have been infusing your water.

Kiwi Water

Makes 8 cups (64 ounces)   Prep time: 3 minutes

Kiwis are often sold several to a bag, so you will have plenty to use in making kiwi-infused water. Using kiwis as an infusion ingredient is both delicious and beautiful due to the bright green color of the fruit. If you use organic kiwis, there is no need to peel the fruit before infusion, but be sure to use a fine strainer to remove pieces of kiwi fuzz floating in your water.

3 or 4 kiwis, peeled
8 cups water

Cut the kiwis into ¼-inch slices and put them in a pitcher.

Muddle the fruit by mashing it with a wooden spoon to create a stronger infusion.

Pour in the water to cover the fruit and chill for 1 to 12 hours before serving.

To absorb iron, you need vitamin C. Pairing Kiwi Water with iron-rich meals can help your body utilize more of this energizing mineral.

Ginger Water

Ginger is terrific to get your blood flowing and your energy up. Unlike ginger tea, ginger-infused water is light with a ginger kick to it. If you are using organic ginger, you probably won't need to peel it—there is no need for that extra step, except for peeling away any pesticide residue from conventional ginger.

3- to 5-inch piece fresh ginger
8 cups water

Slice the ginger and put it in a pitcher.

Pour the water over the ginger pieces and chill for 2 to 12 hours before serving.

One-Step Infusions

Ginger can be reused. Add other ingredients on top of it for a different infusion.

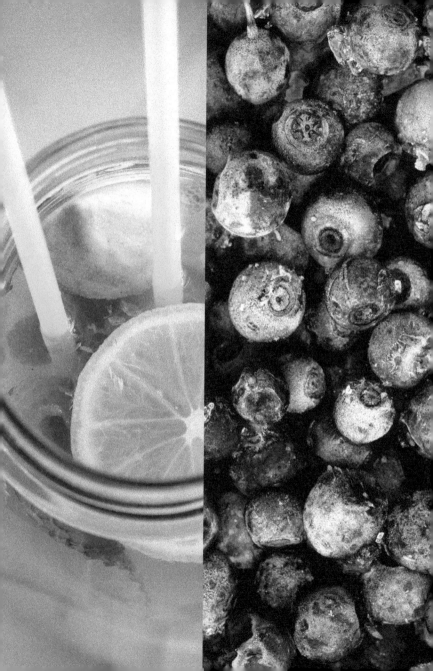

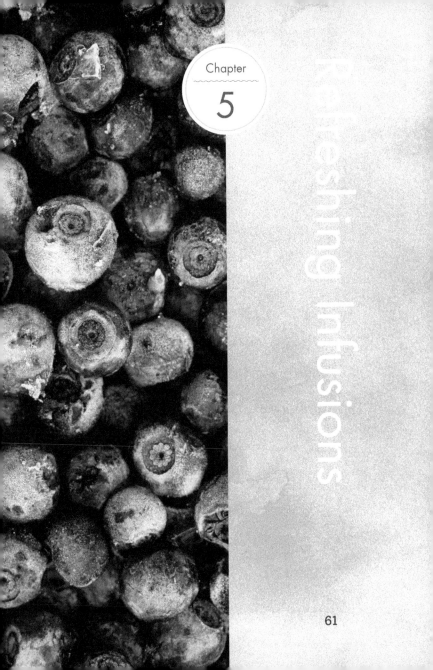

Refreshing Infusions

While all infusions are naturally refreshing due to their water content, the recipes in this chapter are made with special ingredients to give you an extra boost of refreshment that would be welcome on a hot day or after a workout. Imagine yourself relaxing at an exclusive spa as you sip these refreshing infusions, or take them on your next hike through the hills or on a Sunday at the shore.

Remember that the fruit-infused water recipes in this book are just guides to get you started. There is no magic formula to create the perfect infusion that will automatically rehydrate and refresh you in an instant. But the ingredients used in the recipes in this chapter are known for their refreshing qualities, in particular mango, pineapple, and green apple. Mint is naturally uplifting and refreshing, while a hint of rosemary can create a stunning flavor when paired with fresh fruit. Get creative and see what you can come up with after you have played with these recipes for a little while.

Lemon Lime and Mint Infusion

Makes 8 cups (64 ounces)   Prep time: 3 minutes

Lemon, lime, and mint are a terrific combination for just about any occasion. This infusion is beautiful to look at and will put a smile on your guests' faces if you bring it out for gatherings. You might even want to add a touch of your favorite sweetener to create a bright and healthy mint julep treat.

1 or 2 lemons
1 or 2 limes
2 or 3 fresh mint sprigs
4 cups ice cubes
4 cups water

Slice the fruits and put them along with the mint in a pitcher.

Put the ice on top of the ingredients to hold them down and pour the water on top.

Chill for 2 to 8 hours before serving.

This refreshing infusion can be refilled with water and used for a day or two.

Tropical Mango Orange Infusion

Makes 8 cups (64 ounces)   Prep time: 6 minutes

You will feel like you are living on a tropical island while you enjoy this fresh and fruity infused water. This infusion can be refilled with water to enjoy all day long, but after about 24 hours these fruits have given their best and you should start with new ingredients the next day.

1 ripe mango
1 large orange
8 cups water

Peel and pit the mango, then slice it using a sharp knife.

Cut the orange into slices, leaving the peel on.

Put the fruit in your pitcher and cover with water.

Chill for 2 to 8 hours before serving.

To get a strong flavor right away, muddle the fruits before pouring the water over them. Slice down the flat sides first to get as much flesh as you can, then slice those pieces lengthwise to easily remove the peel.

Green Apple and Lime Infusion

Makes 8 cups (64 ounces)   Prep time: 3 minutes

Slightly tart and green, this is a terrifically refreshing infusion. It's one that goes well with workouts, or keeps your brain clear if you have to sit under fluorescent lights all day long. Green apples help keep you hydrated—here they lend just enough sweet and sour flavor to cancel out the lethargy caused by having too much salt in a meal.

1 large or 2 small green apples, sliced
1 or 2 limes, sliced
6 cups ice cubes
2 cups water

Put the sliced fruit in your pitcher and cover with ice.

Pour the water on top.

Chill for 3 to 12 hours before serving.

Remember that you will get the most flavor from hard fruits like apples if you let them infuse for a longer chilling time.

Strawberry Lemon Mint Infusion

Be sure to select sweet and flavorful strawberries to make the most of this infusion. A dark red color and a lack of white flesh around the stem usually indicates a better-tasting strawberry. This infusion can also blend well with sparkling water and a hint of your favorite sweetener.

6 to 10 strawberries, sliced
1 or 2 lemons, sliced
2 fresh mint sprigs
8 cups water

Put the fruit and mint in a pitcher.

Cover with water and chill for 3 to 12 hours before serving.

You may wish to muddle the fruits or bruise the mint to release the flavors before adding the water. You can also crush the mint between your fingers before it adding to your pitcher.

Refreshing Infusions

Cucumber Basil Infusion

Cooling cucumber gets a power boost of refreshment here with the addition of fresh basil. The lightness will almost lift you off your feet. Basil has been known to reduce swelling; coupled with cucumber, it makes a perfect refreshing infusion for any hot day when you're feeling a bit plumped up.

Fruit Infused Water

1 large or 3 small cucumbers, sliced
5 large fresh basil leaves
8 cups water

Put the cucumbers and basil in a pitcher.

Cover the ingredients with water.

Chill for 2 to 12 hours before serving.

You can crush or slice the basil to get more flavor if you wish, but it is good to leave the leaves whole in this recipe to allow the cucumber to stand out.

Rosemary Watermelon Infusion

This refreshing infusion is so elegant that you can keep your pitcher by the pool or give yourself a treat as you study or work. It's good for your brain and for your cells because watermelon, true to its name, is mostly water. This fruit infuses wonderfully and muddles easily, giving over its lovely flavor quite easily. This beverage is the perfect way to enjoy fresh watermelon without overeating and giving yourself the possibility of a bellyache.

Refreshing Infusions

  2 cups watermelon, chopped
  ½ tablespoon fresh rosemary leaves
  8 cups water

Put the watermelon chunks in a pitcher and muddle to release the flavor.

Add the rosemary and water.

Chill for 1 to 12 hours before serving.

Honeydew Orange Basil Infusion

Makes 8 cups (64 ounces)   Prep time: 3–7 minutes

Honeydew is rich in potassium, which is essential for maintaining healthy blood pressure. In this recipe the flavorful honeydew, with its health-boosting benefits, blends perfectly with the fresh and fruity flavors of orange and basil to create a refreshing infused beverage. Enjoy this drink on the porch on a hot summer evening, or keep it in your water bottle to enjoy all day long.

1 orange
2 cups honeydew melon flesh, cut into chunks
3 to 5 large fresh basil leaves
8 cups water

Put the fruits in a pitcher.

Muddle with a wooden spoon or muddler, then add the basil and water.

Chill for 1 to 12 hours before serving.

When choosing a honeydew, be sure to pick one that is heavy for its size, with outer skin that looks more waxy than fuzzy. Avoid melons that are bruised and those that do not bounce back when pressed.

Blueberry Lemon Infusion

Makes 8 cups (64 ounces)   Prep time: 3 minutes

Blueberries seem to taste sweeter when there is lemon nearby—try it the next time you make blueberry pie. You could add sweetener to this infusion if you like, but see how refreshing it is with the hint of blueberry and zip of lemon.

- 1 to 2 cups fresh blueberries
- 1 lemon, sliced
- 8 cups water

Put the blueberries into a pitcher and muddle gently with a wooden spoon or muddler.

Add the lemon slices and water.

Chill for 1 to 12 hours before serving.

Grapefruit Vanilla Infusion

Tart grapefruit with fragrant vanilla could be a dessert or a breakfast, but it is delightfully refreshing as an infusion. Feel free to add a hint of sweetness with stevia or your preferred sweetener—a touch of honey can also be delicious. When prepared without added sweetener, this grapefruit and vanilla–infused water may help curb your appetite.

1 vanilla bean
1 grapefruit, sliced
8 cups water

Put the vanilla bean in a pitcher and muddle if desired.

Add the grapefruit slices and the water.

Chill for 2 to 12 hours before serving.

Mandarin Ginger Infusion

Makes 8 cups (64 ounces)   Prep time: 5 minutes

This refreshing infusion combines the fresh flavor of mandarin oranges with the health benefits of ginger in one delicious beverage that is sure to brighten up your day. Use as much fresh ginger as you like for a strong taste, or leave the recipe as is for a gentle infusion that is both sweet and spicy.

2 or 3 mandarin oranges, sliced
2-inch piece fresh ginger, sliced
8 cups water

Put the mandarin slices and ginger in a pitcher.

Muddle the ingredients, if desired, then add the water.

Chill for 1 to 12 hours before serving.

If you want a very gingery infusion, you can grate the ginger instead of slicing it, but be sure to use a sieve or strainer to catch the juice.

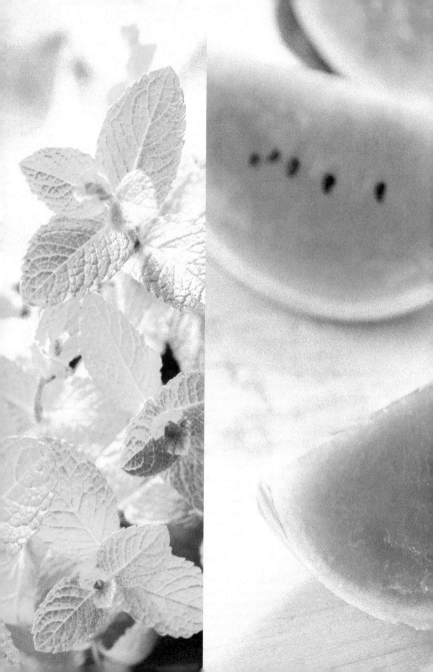

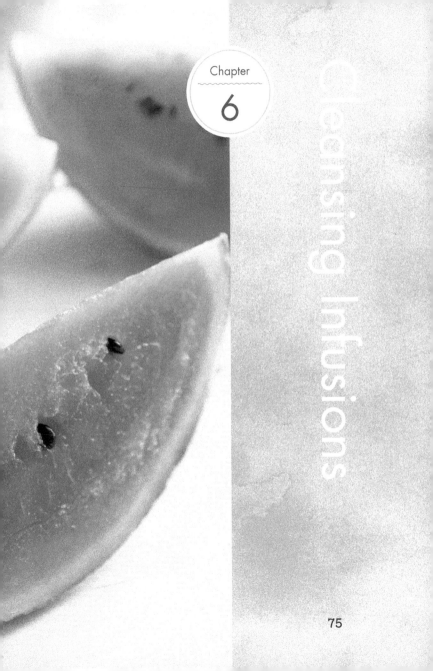

Chapter

6

Cleansing Infusions

Many fruits are known for their cleansing and detoxifying properties, largely due to their high levels of water and antioxidants. Cleansing involves helping the body eliminate toxins and clear away impurities. Drinking plenty of water is essential for this function because it helps flush out accumulated toxins, which helps purify the body. To avoid putting any new toxins into your body as you cleanse, purchase organically grown ingredients. This will ensure that you are getting the cleansing benefits you want without any residues, waxes, or chemicals that are often found in commercially grown produce.

The infusions presented in this chapter are the perfect complement to a healthy diet. However, these recipes are not meant to be used as a cleanse. If you plan to engage in a juice or herbal cleanse, be sure to check with your health-care professional to ensure that you are not mixing items that could interact poorly due to a health condition. Use these infusions as healthy, delicious drinks that just happen to offer a bit of cleansing for gentle detoxification along with your daily hydration.

Parsley Lemon Infusion

Makes 8 cups (64 ounces)   Prep time: 3 minutes

Parsley has a fresh and vibrant taste that works surprisingly well as an infusion ingredient, giving an earthy tone to the sourness of lemon. This is a supercleansing combination that is also alkalizing and good for your breath.

2 lemons, sliced
4 or 5 fresh parsley sprigs
6 cups ice cubes
2 cups water

Put the lemons and parsley in a pitcher and pour the ice on top.

Pour in the water and chill for 1 to 12 hours before serving.

You may crush the parsley leaves before adding them to the pitcher if you want a richer flavor and deeper benefits for your infusion. You may choose to muddle the lemon slices as well.

Apple Ginger Infusion

Makes 8 cups (64 ounces)   Prep time: 4 minutes

Both apple and ginger are good for digestion and can help the body gently eliminate toxins. Infusing these ingredients into water can have a subtle detoxifying effect, and it tastes delicious as well. Do not be afraid to use apples that might be a little soft—infusing them will bring out their flavor and you will not have to worry about their texture.

2 apples, sliced (any variety)
2-inch piece fresh ginger, sliced
8 cups water

Put the apple and ginger slices in a pitcher.

Muddle for a minute or two then pour the water on top.

Chill for 2 to 12 hours before serving.

Use organic apples to avoid the pesticides that often linger on commercially grown fruits. Conventional apples are usually at the top of the "dirty dozen" list for having more than 40 different chemicals detected on them by the time they are picked. If you are not sure if the apples you are looking at are organic, check the code on the sticker. If it starts with a 4, it is conventionally grown; if it starts with a 9, it is organic.

Cranberry Lime Basil Infusion

Makes 8 cups (64 ounces)   Prep time: 8 minutes

Cleansing cranberries are enhanced by lively lime to produce a great infusion for any time of year. This beverage is also a perfect red-and-green combination to serve at holiday gatherings.

½ cup fresh cranberries
2 limes, sliced
6 cups ice cubes
2 cups water

Pierce the cranberries carefully with the tip of a knife and put them in a pitcher.

Add the sliced limes and pour the ice on top of the fruit.

Pour in the water and chill for 1 to 12 hours before serving.

Lavender Lemon Infusion

Makes 8 cups (64 ounces)   Prep time: 2 minutes

You might not think of lavender as an ingredient for beverages, but it is just as delicious in infusions as it is in shortbread cookies. This herb is soothing when paired with lovely lemon for a new twist on a cleansing beverage.

1 tablespoon culinary lavender
2 or 3 lemons, sliced
6 cups ice cubes
2 cups water

Put the lavender in a pitcher with the lemon slices on top. Put the ice on top of the lemons, then pour in the water. Chill for 1 to 12 hours before serving.

Remember to purchase lavender that has not been sprayed, dyed, or treated in any way. Organic culinary lavender can often be found at farmers' markets, or you might want to grow your own.

Cinnamon Peach Infusion

Sweet peaches pair wonderfully with cinnamon in a cobbler, pie, crisp, smoothie, or infusion. The only cleansing way to enjoy this dynamic combo is in a simple infusion, like this one, that you can enjoy all day long if you wish.

Fruit Infused Water

2 or 3 ripe peaches, pitted and sliced
1 cinnamon stick
8 cups water

Put the peaches in a pitcher and muddle for 1 minute.

Add the cinnamon stick and water.

Chill for 1 to 12 hours before serving.

Strawberry Grapefruit Sage Infusion

Makes 8 cups (64 ounces)   Prep time: 5 minutes

This is a unique flavor combination that is both cleansing and calming. If you love grapefruit, then you will enjoy a water giving you the benefits of grapefruit with a bit of sweetness from the strawberries and a lovely twist of sage.

1 grapefruit, sliced
1 cup fresh strawberries, sliced
4 fresh sage leaves
8 cups water

Put the grapefruit and strawberries in a pitcher.

Add the sage and water, then chill for 1 to 12 hours before serving.

If you wish to gently muddle the ingredients, wait until you drink the infusion and refill the water—if you muddle from the beginning and reuse the ingredients you will mostly taste the sage.

Fig Orange Lavender Infusion

Makes 8 cups (64 ounces)   Prep time: 5 minutes

Figs and oranges are a very sweet combination for a lovely flavor. This recipe uses just a touch of lavender, but you can use more if you want to. Slicing the fruits and letting the fruit and lavender sit in the water will look better than muddling and mashing, but if you would rather muddle for flavor, you can skip slicing the figs if they are very ripe.

4 ripe figs, sliced
2 oranges, sliced
1 teaspoon culinary lavender
8 cups water

Put the figs, oranges, and lavender in a pitcher.

Cover with water and chill for 1 to 12 hours before serving.

If you don't want to have to strain your infusions when using a pitcher or a jar that isn't specially designed for making infusions, you can also put the ingredients into a cheesecloth bag. This will not give you as strong an infusion, but it will save you the hassle of straining.

Basil Lemon Lime Infusion

Makes 8 cups (64 ounces)   Prep time: 5 minutes

Basil is a versatile herb that provides powerful cleansing benefits in fusion with lemon and lime. Known as a restorative herb, basil makes this infusion both cleansing and restorative—it can be a good one if you are feeling fatigued.

    5 large fresh basil leaves
    2 lemons, sliced
    1 lime, sliced
    8 cups water

Crush the basil leaves with your fingers, then add them to your pitcher.

Add the rest of the ingredients and chill for 1 to 8 hours before serving.

Watermelon Grape Infusion

Makes 8 cups (64 ounces)   Prep time: 6 minutes

Use either green or red grapes for this infusion. Green grapes combined with the red watermelon make for an attractive presentation, but both kinds of grapes will have a flavorful effect. Grapes have a high sugar content and not as much fiber as other fruits, so both grapes and watermelon muddle easily to release their essence into your water.

10 grapes, halved
2 cups watermelon, cut into chunks
8 cups water

Put the grapes and watermelon into a pitcher and muddle for 1 minute.

Pour the water over the fruit and chill for 1 to 8 hours before serving.

Frozen grapes are a fun summer treat. Pop any grapes you have left over after preparing this recipe into the freezer to enjoy later.

Kiwi Apple Infusion

Makes 8 cups (64 ounces)   Prep time: 5 minutes

Be sure to use ripe kiwis for this recipe—the fruit should gently give when you press on it. Do not worry if the kiwis look like they have water spots on their skin. As one of the most nutrient-dense fruits, kiwis often don't get the attention they deserve, but they are great coupled with the ever-popular apple for a delightful and cleansing infusion.

2 apples, sliced
3 or 4 kiwis, peeled and sliced
8 cups of water

Put the apples into your pitcher and muddle for a minute or two.

Add the kiwis and cover with water.

Chill for 2 to 12 hours before serving.

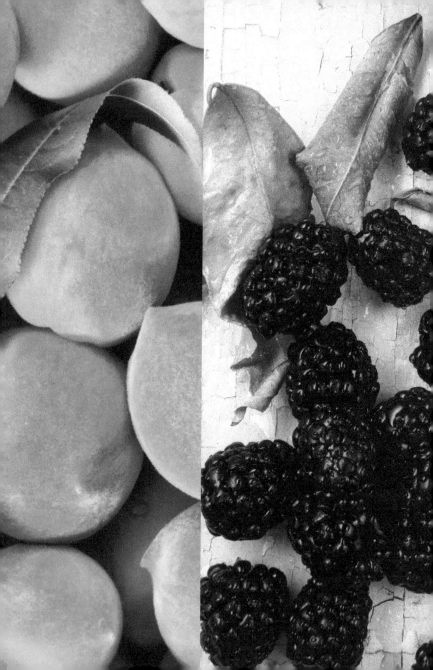

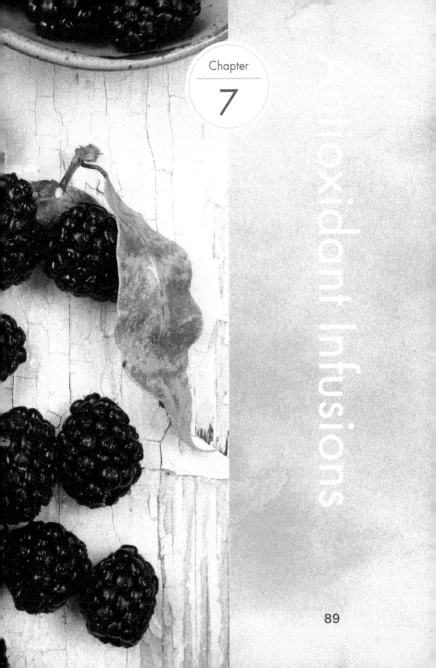

Chapter

7

Antioxidant Infusions

Antioxidants are substances found in food that can help protect your cells against certain kinds of damage. While some antioxidants are artificial, the most powerful come from natural food sources like fruits and leafy greens. Antioxidants may protect you from certain types of cancer and other diseases by preventing oxidation in the cells. Oxidation (like rust on metal) is a process that produces free radicals, which can break down your cells and impact your health, so eating antioxidant-rich foods gives your cells the protection they need to keep your youthful looks and vibrant energy.

While you can take dietary supplements to increase your intake of antioxidants, it is generally safer to increase your intake by eating antioxidant-rich foods. Antioxidants like beta-carotene, lutein, lycopene, selenium, and vitamins A, C, and E can be found in a variety of foods. Some fruits are among the most antioxidant-rich foods available, including blueberries, cranberries, apples, plums, cherries, and strawberries. You will find these ingredients and more in the antioxidant infusion recipes in this chapter.

Chile Water

Makes 8 cups (64 ounces)   Prep time: 2 minutes

Capsaicin in chiles is a compound that is so good for your heart and circulatory system that herbalists claim it can prevent a heart attack. At the very least, it can definitely stir up the circulation of your blood. You can control the heat and flavor of this infusion by how you slice your peppers. Not slicing them at all can give you just a hint of flavor while slicing them fine might be a tad too pungent to enjoy. If you have chronic bronchial problems or just want to protect your cells, a middle-of-the-road approach might be best.

1 or 2 chiles, sliced
8 cups water

Put the chiles in a pitcher.

Pour the water over the chiles and chill for 2 to 12 hours before serving.

Blackberry Orange Water

Makes 8 cups (64 ounces)   Prep time: 5 minutes

Blackberries and oranges not only look pretty together, but their flavors combine as if they were mixed by Merlin himself. This is a magical elixir high in vitamin C and antioxidants. Blackberry Orange Water might even lure the object of your attention to you, just so they could keep enjoying this sultry sweet combo.

1 cup fresh blackberries
1 or 2 oranges, sliced
8 cups water

Put the berries and orange slices in a pitcher.

Muddle the ingredients for 2 minutes.

Add the water and chill for 1 to 8 hours before serving.

If you don't have a long-handled wooden spoon or a muddler, use any item that you have in your kitchen—even a potato masher. Muddle gently if you just want the flavor to be light, but many people enjoy a well-muddled infusion. Portable infusers often have a turning compartment to muddle the ingredients, and some infusion pitchers come with a muddler that specifically fits the center infusion tube.

Plum Mint and Lime Water

High in antioxidants, plums go great with common spearmint and lime to produce a classy, healthy infused water that is fun to drink. You might even find it more refreshing than lemonade.

- 4 ripe plums, pitted and sliced
- 1 or 2 limes, sliced
- 3 fresh mint sprigs
- 8 cups water

Put the plum and lime slices in a pitcher.

Muddle for a minute if you wish.

Crush or rub the mint leaves between your fingers and add to the pitcher.

Pour the water on top and chill for 1 to 12 hours before serving.

If you wish to add a touch of sweetener such as stevia to this infusion, wait until after it has infused to add it and get the flavor right for your taste.

Fruit Infused Water

Apricot Nectarine Rosemary Water

Makes 8 cups (64 ounces)   Prep time: 4 minutes

The sweetness of ripe nectarines and apricots paired with a hint of rosemary is a unique infusion experience. Apricot season is short and prized because a fresh, just-off-the-tree fruit is exceptional.

    4 ripe apricots, pitted and sliced
    2 or 3 ripe nectarines, pitted and sliced
    1 teaspoon fresh rosemary leaves
    8 cups water

Put the apricots and nectarines in a pitcher with the rosemary.

Muddle the ingredients for a minute or two.

Add the water and chill for 2 to 8 hours before serving.

Be sure to let your fruit ripen before using them in this infusion, or the flavor will be flat.

Cherry Vanilla Water

Makes 8 cups (64 ounces)   Prep time: 9 minutes

This antioxidant-rich infusion is a great one to help you relive the days of classic soda-shop beverages. The flavors in this recipe pair well, and once they are infused they are light and peppy. This infusion can be made with sparkling water as well.

1 vanilla bean
1½ to 2 cups fresh cherries, pitted
8 cups water

Put the vanilla bean into the pitcher and crush slightly with a muddler.

Add the cherries, then muddle the ingredients for a minute.

Pour in the water, then chill for 1 to 8 hours before serving.

If you are using a cherry pitter to remove the pits from your cherries, you may want to slice your cherries in half after pitting them. If you are removing the pits with a knife, your fruits will already be sliced and you can just toss them into your pitcher.

Cranberry Peach Water

Makes 8 cups (64 ounces)   Prep time: 9 minutes

Both cranberries and peaches are high in antioxidants, and their flavors complement each other well. When you can't find peaches, you might also enjoy cranberries paired with orange. Smooth and satiating, Cranberry Peach Water is an easy one to keep sipping.

1 cup fresh or frozen cranberries
2 or 3 ripe peaches, pitted and sliced
8 cups water

Pierce each cranberry to let out the flavor and put them in a pitcher.

Add the peaches, then cover with water.

Chill for 2 to 8 hours before serving.

If you are using frozen cranberries, do not pierce them before adding them to the pitcher. You can successfully use dried cranberries in this recipe as an alternative to the fresh or frozen fruit, but be sure to buy unsweetened dried cranberries. If you can't find unsweetened ones, use apple-sweetened dried cranberries and use ⅓ to ½ cup instead of a whole cup.

Mixed Melon Sage Water

Makes 8 cups (64 ounces)   Prep time: 2–7 minutes

Watermelon, true to its name, is mostly composed of water and is delightfully sweet. Sage seems to bring out a flavor twist that is just right, provided you go easy on the herb and strong on the melon. Other melons pair up nicely with sage and can be combined any way you choose. You can buy your melons precut for fast infusions, or simply slice them into wedges and cut the flesh away from the rind—no need to make perfect cubes or balls unless you are concerned about presentation.

3 large sage leaves
1 cup watermelon, chopped
1 cup cantaloupe or other melon, chopped
8 cups water

Put the sage leaves in a pitcher and muddle.

Add the melons and muddle, if you like.

Add the water and chill for 1 to 12 hours before serving.

Blueberry Apple Water

Makes 8 cups (64 ounces)   Prep time: 3 minutes

Apples and blueberries go nicely together to make a sweet and tart infusion—they also pair well with cinnamon and lemon if you wish to add either of those ingredients. Both fruits are high in antioxidants; blueberries in particular have antiviral properties. Blueberries are also thought to be good for memory.

- 2 red apples, sliced
- 1 cup fresh blueberries
- 8 cups water

Put the apples in your pitcher.

Muddle for a minute or two.

Add the blueberries and muddle gently.

Add the water and chill for 1 to 12 hours before serving.

You do not need to core the apples before using them in your infusions. Seeds can be bitter, however, so to get a sweeter infusion with this recipe, remove the seeds before slicing.

Red Grape
Kiwi Water

Makes 8 cups (64 ounces)   Prep time: 6 minutes

Red grapes and kiwis are beautiful to look at in your water pitcher and they are high in antioxidant goodness. Like a fruity wine infusion, this beverage gives you a pleasingly sweet and tangy infusion with an exotic taste.

3 ripe kiwis, peeled
1 cup red seedless grapes
8 cups water

Put the kiwis and grapes in a pitcher.

Muddle for a minute if you wish.

Add the water and chill for 2 to 10 hours before serving.

Fruit Infused Water

Mango Apricot Chile Water

Makes 8 cups (64 ounces)　Prep time: 5 minutes

A touch of chile gives this infusion a south-of-the-border taste. The spiciness wakes up the sweet fruits and brings them to life. No wonder mangoes find their way into salads and savory dishes as well as sweet ones!

- 1 ripe mango, peeled, pitted, and sliced
- 3 ripe apricots, pitted and sliced
- 1 fresh chile or 1 pinch cayenne pepper
- 8 cups water

Put the mango and apricot in a pitcher.

Muddle for a minute if you wish.

Add the chile or pinch of cayenne pepper.

Add the water and chill for 2 to 12 hours before serving.

When washing or handling chiles, people with sensitive skin might want to wear gloves. Surgical gloves are a great kitchen tool to keep fingers from getting stained with herbs such as turmeric, or irritated when handling items such as peppers.

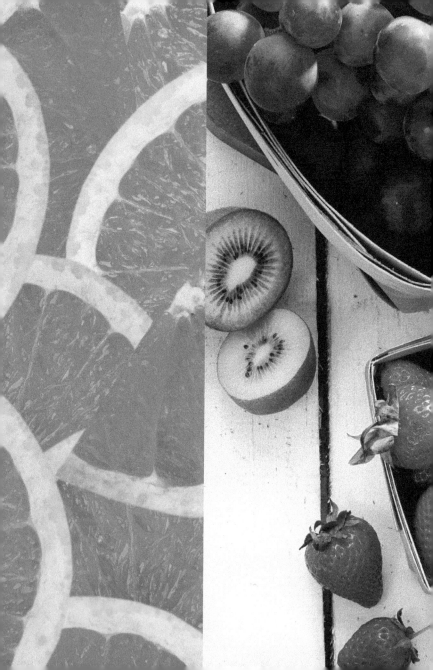

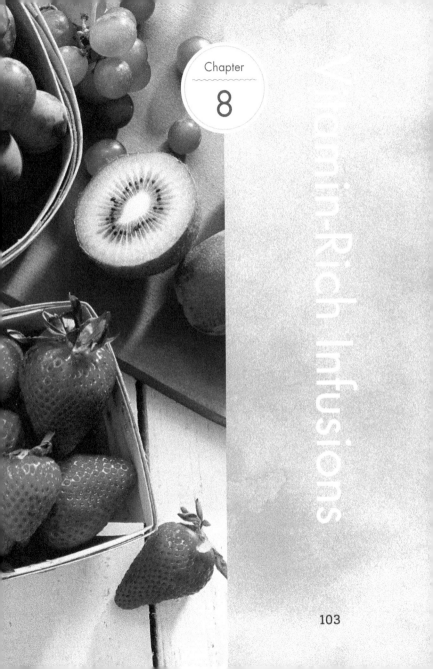

Chapter

8

Vitamin-Rich Infusions

While taking vitamin supplements is a fairly common practice, it may not be the most efficient way to increase your vitamin intake. The truth of the matter is that your body cannot absorb vitamins from supplements as readily as it can those from natural food sources. When you drink a vitamin-rich fruit infusion, your body can absorb and utilize the vitamins more easily than it can with any supplement. While science has not yet determined the exact vitamin content water absorbs during infusion as compared to eating whole fruits, you can be certain that the infusions in this chapter offer a simple way to increase your vitamin intake without the sugar load that you get from juicing or drinking smoothies.

While both juices and smoothies have nutritional benefits and can be considered healthy treats, these infusions can be enjoyed in greater quantities due to their low calorie impact. Remember that just because your infusion provides extra vitamins, it is not a substitute for eating well and following the recommendations of your physician. These vitamin-rich fruit infusions are fun to drink and provide an extra nutrient boost to your already healthful lifestyle.

Raspberry Peach Pineapple Infusion

Makes 8 cups (64 ounces)   Prep time: 5 minutes

Thiamine, niacin, and wonderful pantothenic acid, great for the skin, are all infused into this delicious water. Raspberry and pineapple both provide folic acid, and of course, you get vitamins C and E and even some vitamin K. These fruits are easy infusers and mingle nicely together. Healthy does taste great!

1 cup fresh raspberries
2 peaches, pitted and sliced
1 cup pineapple chunks
8 cups water

Put the fruits into a pitcher and muddle for a minute.

Add the water and chill for 1 to 8 hours before serving.

If you purchased a fresh whole pineapple, be sure it is fragrant and that you can easily pull out one of the top leaves to make sure it is ripe. Then just cut away the rind and use the sweet yellow flesh.

Grapefruit Watermelon Infusion

High in vitamins A, C, and B, this Grapefruit Watermelon Infusion is an energizing and slenderizing duo. The sweetness of watermelon tames the bitter tones of the grapefruit to give you an infusion that is packed with vitamins and lovely to sip on. To enhance the flavor, you might consider adding a bit of herb such as mint or basil. Try it in varying amounts to get the taste that pleases you most.

    1 grapefruit, sliced
    2 cups watermelon, chopped
    8 cups water

Put the fruit into a pitcher and muddle for a minute.

Add water and chill for 1 to 8 hours before serving.

Blackberry Pear Infusion

Makes 8 cups (64 ounces)   Prep time: 7 minutes

This is a luscious combination that looks beautiful in a jar or pitcher. Blackberries have vitamins A and C and some B vitamins as well. Pear has A, C, and B vitamins and a bit of vitamin E. Both can help rid the body of environmental toxins.

1 large or 2 small pears
1 to 2 cups fresh blackberries
8 cups water

Slice the pear, leaving the core behind, and put in a pitcher.

Muddle for a minute to release the flavor, then add the blackberries.

Muddle for a minute more.

Add the water and chill for 1 to 12 hours before serving.

Need to speed up the ripening process for your fruits? Put them in a paper bag and set it in warm spot in your kitchen. During winter months, the top of your refrigerator might be the warmest spot.

Banana Mango Peach Infusion

Makes 8 cups (64 ounces)   Prep time: 3 minutes

Sweet, fruity, and vitamin-rich, this is a tropical infusion that makes drinking water seem like a treat. This infusion works nicely with lavender or basil as well. A peach has 6 micrograms of folate along with a far higher content of vitamins A, C, and K. Banana has a surprising 10.3 milligrams of vitamin C along with its high potassium content, as well as B vitamins and a bit of vitamins A and E. Mango has a higher vitamin content than banana, so all in all, you'll quench your thirst and be nourished from this sweet infusion.

1 ripe banana, sliced
1 ripe mango, peeled, pitted, and sliced
2 ripe peaches, pitted and sliced
6 cups ice cubes
2 cups water

Put the fruit slices into a pitcher and muddle for a minute.

Put the ice on top of the fruits and add the water.

Chill for 1 to 12 hours before serving.

Strawberry Watermelon Mint Infusion

Makes 8 cups (64 ounces)   Prep time: 3 minutes

Vitamin A and folate can be found in all three ingredients in this recipe. Strawberries and watermelon are not just a sweet combination; they also provide some of the highest vitamin contents found in fruits. This fruity infusion is popular with those who have never had a water infusion before—and it looks pretty, too!

2 fresh mint sprigs
1½ cups sliced strawberries
2 cups watermelon chunks
8 cups water

Put the mint sprigs in a pitcher and muddle.

Add the fruits and muddle for a minute.

Add the water and chill for 1 to 8 hours before serving.

To keep this infusion fresh and fruity all day long, you can add some sliced fruit to it each time the water level goes down and then add more water to fill it back up.

Grape Banana Orange Infusion

High in vitamin A, grapes also have 22 micrograms of vitamin K, which keeps bones healthy. This vitamin-packed trio of ingredients yields a fun infusion that will remind you of summertime even when the leaves have left the trees.

- 1 or 2 oranges, sliced
- 1 cup green seedless grapes
- 1 ripe banana, peeled and sliced
- 8 cups water

Put the orange slices into a pitcher and muddle a little.

Add the grapes and muddle a bit more.

Add the banana and pour in the water.

Chill for 2 to 12 hours before serving.

If you have a bunch of bananas that are getting too ripe, peel them and freeze the fruit for infusions, smoothies, and snacks. They will last in your freezer for several months.

Pineapple Strawberry Grape Infusion

Makes 8 cups (64 ounces)   Prep time: 3 minutes

This is another vitamin-rich combination that is sweet and flavorful. Strawberry and pineapple go well together, plus you get a distinctive musky flavor from the grapes. Use red or green grapes in this recipe, and for an even bigger vitamin C punch, add lemon slices to the mix.

- 1 cup pineapple chunks
- 1 cup sliced strawberries
- 1 cup green or red seedless grapes
- 8 cups water

Put the fruits into a pitcher and muddle for a minute.

Add the water and chill for 1 to 8 hours before serving.

Kiwi Raspberry Infusion

Makes 8 cups (64 ounces)   Prep time: 3 minutes

Kiwis are packed with vitamin C, vitamin A, B vitamins, and vitamin K. While the acidity of oranges can upset the stomach for some people, kiwis are mild enough that they typically don't cause a problem. Paired with juicy raspberries, the kiwis in this recipe make for a terrific immunity-boosting infusion.

- 1½ cups fresh raspberries
- 3 kiwis, peeled and sliced
- 8 cups water

Put the fruit into a pitcher and muddle for a minute or two.

Add the water and chill for 1 to 8 hours before serving.

Parsley Lime Peach Infusion

Makes 8 cups (64 ounces)   Prep time: 3 minutes

Parsley is not only extremely high in vitamins A and C, it also has a lot of iron and calcium. Infused with lime and peach, this salad green turns into a beautiful beverage.

2 limes, sliced
3 peaches, pitted and sliced
3 or 4 fresh parsley sprigs
6 cups ice cubes
2 cups water

Put the limes in a pitcher, and then put the peach slices on top.

Muddle for a minute, and then add the parsley with the ice on top.

Pour in the water and let the mixture infuse for 3 to 12 hours before serving.

You can muddle the parsley if you wish, but only if you want the parsley essence to stand out beyond the other ingredients. Muddling the fruits and letting the parsley infuse gently creates a more balanced blend of the ingredients.

Summer Berry Blast Infusion

Makes 8 cups (64 ounces)   Prep time: 3 minutes

Strawberries, blueberries, and blackberries all signify various months of summertime. Pick your own when you can and freeze some ripe berries for when they are no longer available. If you find yourself out of strawberries, use raspberries for this vitamin- and antioxidant-rich infusion.

- 1 cup fresh blueberries
- 1 cup fresh blackberries
- 1 cup sliced strawberries
- 8 cups water

Put the berries into a pitcher and muddle for 1 minute.

Add the water and chill for 1 to 8 hours before serving.

Washing berries usually involves rinsing the berries in a strainer under water. You can also use a vegetable wash that comes in a spray bottle, if you wish. The fine mist is easy to rinse off and it gives many people ease of mind, knowing that their berries are clean.

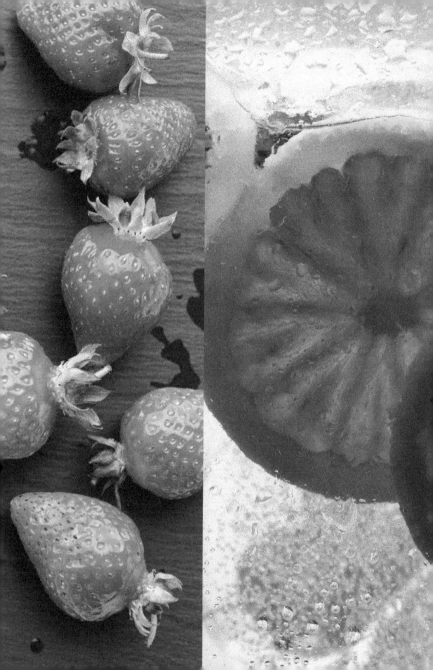

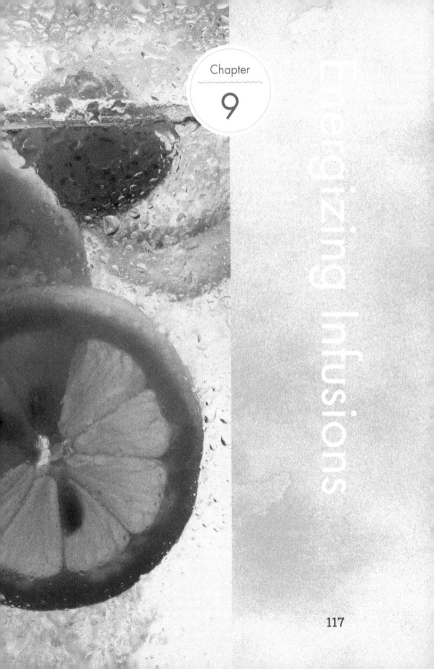

Chapter

9

Energizing Infusions

F ruit infusions are intrinsically energizing because they are loaded with healthy vitamins and minerals. Getting good hydration from fresh fruits also helps improve your energy level, and since most fruits are high in vitamins A and C, they also help your immunity. If your body is working hard to fight off a cold or infection, it can use up your immediate energy reserves and slow you down. These energizing infusions are made with energy-rich ingredients that will replenish those stores and leave you feeling strong. Many of the ingredients used in these recipes also contain B vitamins, which directly contribute to the production of ATP, the source of your cellular energy.

For your body to be functioning at its highest level with good energy, it needs to be balanced—the ideal pH for your body is slightly alkaline. Have you ever felt a boost of energy and improved mental clarity after drinking highly alkalized water? Eating well and maintaining your body's pH balance gives you that feeling every day. These energizing infusions won't get you buzzing like coffee, but they will give you clean, clear, and healthy energy, which is something you might like even better.

Apricot Lemon Infusion

Makes 8 cups (64 ounces)   Prep time: 3 minutes

Ripe, golden-orange apricots mix so well with lemons that you might want to buy extra to make an apricot lemon pudding or pie, or just to eat apricots spritzed with lemon while you sip on this energizing infusion. Apricots can ease dryness in your skin and hair—they are a special summer fruit.

    4 or 5 apricots, pitted and sliced
    2 lemons, sliced
    8 cups water

Put the apricots in a pitcher with the lemons.

Muddle for a minute, then add the water.

Chill for 1 to 8 hours before serving.

Blueberry Mango Lime Infusion

Makes 8 cups (64 ounces)   Prep time: 6 minutes

Delicious alkalizing lime brings out the sweetness of the blueberries and mango. If you have ever thought about getting more color into your diet, the green, blue, and orange hues of this trio are a wonderful way to start—they look great in the pitcher, too.

1 mango, peeled, pitted, and cut into chunks
1 cup fresh blueberries
1 or 2 limes, sliced
8 cups water

Put the mango and blueberries in a pitcher.

Muddle for a minute or two.

Add the lime slices and water.

Chill for 1 to 12 hours before serving.

Remember always to pick through your berries before using them in a recipe, to remove any that are rotten or smashed. This will ensure that your infusion is as fresh and flavorful as possible.

Peppermint Peach Infusion

Just thinking about peppermint can give you a slight energy boost. Peppermint and peach are an unusual and uplifting infusion to brighten your day. The energy boost starts the moment you smell the peppermint, triggering a reaction in your brain. You might pocket a leaf when you make this infusion and keep it nearby for a minty aroma anytime you need a little lift.

2 or 3 fresh peppermint sprigs
2 large peaches, pitted and sliced
8 cups water

Put the peppermint in a pitcher and muddle gently.

Add the peach slices and muddle a little more.

Add the water and chill for 2 to 12 hours before serving.

Fruit Infused Water

Ginger Lemon Mango Infusion

Makes 8 cups (64 ounces)   Prep time: 3 minutes

Invigorating ginger pairs up great with sweet mango and sprightly lime for an energizing and uplifting infusion so good you might find it on a menu someday. Ginger tea is a common drink in warm Indonesia, where it is taken to refresh after a journey or on a hot day.

1 ripe mango, peeled, pitted, and sliced
1 or 2 lemons, sliced
2-inch piece fresh ginger, sliced
8 cups water

Put the mango and lemon slices in a pitcher.

Muddle for a minute and add the ginger and the water.

Chill for 1 to 8 hours before serving.

If you have ever heard the expression "thick skin," it can also apply to lemons. If you have trouble finding them organic, don't worry too much. Their thick skin helps keep pesticides and environmental toxins from reaching the inner fruit, and their skin is easy to wash before slicing.

Strawberry Citrus Infusion

Makes 8 cups (64 ounces)   Prep time: 4 minutes

Strawberries are known for their calming scent, but as a lightly sweet fruit that is high in vitamin C, they are also great in an energy infusion paired with citrus fruits. In this recipe you get to choose which citrus fruits you want to infuse—all of them will work. Get the power of lemons and limes for energizing, or the superpower of grapefruit to help with blood sugar and cravings that could slow you down.

1 cup sliced strawberries
1 grapefruit or orange (or 2 lemons or limes), sliced
8 cups water

Put the fruit into a pitcher and muddle for 1 minute if you wish.

Add the water and chill for 1 to 8 hours before serving.

Lemon Vanilla Infusion

Makes 8 cups (64 ounces)   Prep time: 3 minutes

Lemon and vanilla create a light and invigorating mingle of both aroma and taste. It is reminiscent of lemon pie, but far more thirst-quenching and energizing. If you have ever noticed that when you are in a better mood, your energy is higher, then this is an infusion you might like. Vanilla can lift your mood and is said to be able to dissolve pent-up anger. No wonder it is such a prevalent ingredient in perfume and dessert.

1 vanilla bean
3 lemons, sliced
8 cups water

Put the vanilla bean in a pitcher and muddle or crush slightly.

Add the lemons and water.

Chill for 1 to 8 hours before serving.

Lemon Cucumber Parsley Infusion

Makes 8 cups (64 ounces)   Prep time: 3 minutes

Light and full of vitamins and minerals, this trio is earthy instead of sweet. If you want energy from the power of vitamin C mixed with iron and uplifting coolness from the cucumber, this can be a satisfying infusion.

2 or 3 fresh parsley sprigs
1 medium cucumber, sliced
1 or 2 lemons, sliced
8 cups water

Put the parsley, cucumbers, and lemons into a pitcher and muddle if you wish.

Add the water and chill for 2 to 8 hours before serving.

Cinnamon Pear Infusion

Cinnamon and pears go together like the notes of a symphony. The sweet pears blend perfectly with the spicy cinnamon to give you a lovely beverage. Cinnamon's energizing power comes from aiding digestion, and it is also touted as stimulating all of the vital functions of the body, increasing your overall vitality.

- 2 ripe pears, pitted and sliced
- 1 cinnamon stick
- 8 cups water

Put the fruit slices in a pitcher and muddle for 1 minute.

Add the cinnamon stick and water.

Chill for 2 to 12 hours before serving.

If you do not have a cinnamon stick, ground cinnamon will work as well. Organic cinnamon varies in taste, but the taste will show up in your beverage while you are drinking it.

Kiwi Lemon Lime Apple Infusion

Makes 8 cups (64 ounces)   Prep time: 6 minutes

The rule of three can be broken to good effect from time to time. In this recipe kiwi adds a powerful punch of vitamin C, coupled with both lemon and lime that will brighten any day. Apple adds sweetness and a tasty mingling of flavors. This infusion is not only energizing but very thirst-quenching as well.

1 large apple, cored and sliced
2 or 3 kiwis, sliced
1 lemon, sliced
1 lime, sliced
8 cups water

Put all of the fruit into a pitcher.

Muddle for a minute if you wish.

Add the water and chill for 1 to 8 hours before serving.

Strawberry Cocoa Mango Infusion

Makes 8 cups (64 ounces)   Prep time: 3 minutes

Cocoa is naturally energy-boosting due to its caffeine content, but it also adds a peppy note to sweet mango with strawberries. Try to find ripe strawberries, not only to maximize the energizing power of the fruit but also to make the flavor stand out and combine with the mango and cocoa. This is a combination that will put a spring in your step and, of course, a grin on your face.

    ½ teaspoon cocoa powder
    1 ripe mango, peeled, pitted, and sliced
    1 cup sliced strawberries
    8 cups water

Put the cocoa powder in a pitcher.

Put the mango chunks or slices on top and muddle if desired.

Add the strawberries and water.

Chill for 1 to 8 hours before serving.

You can use carob powder as an alternative to cocoa powder. Carob is sweet on its own (rather than bitter, like cocoa) and has no caffeine.

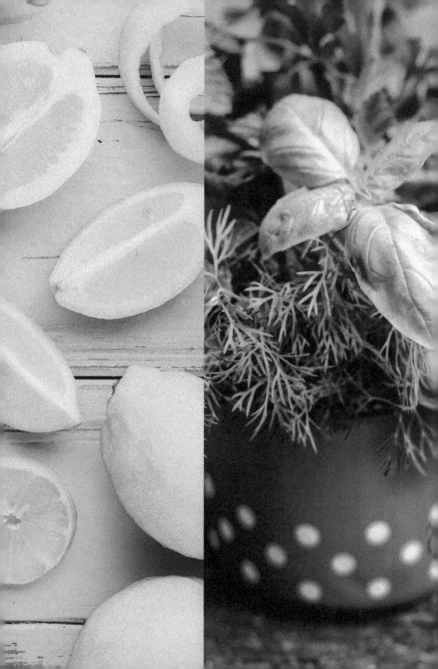

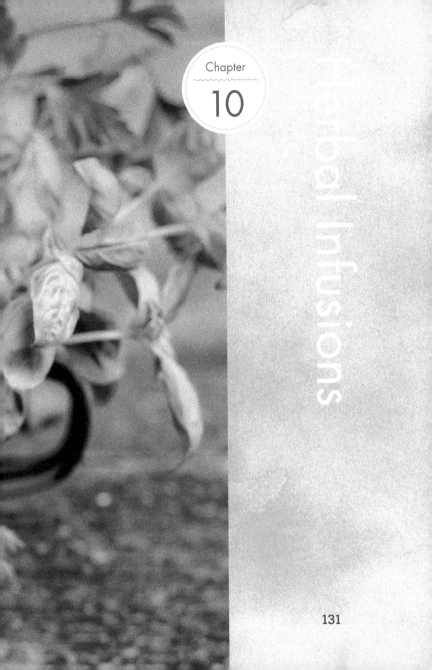

Chapter

10

Herbal Infusions

Sometimes you crave the rich earthy tones of herbal infusions, or you want the medicinal benefits that herbs provide. Herbs are delicious alone or combined, and are quite refreshing and invigorating when used as infusions.

Tea is also an infusion. Tea infusions create a strong herbal beverage that can be too robust for some people, who prefer the gentle aromatics of cold infusions. One great thing about herbal infusions is that they are generally safe for everyone, and they make water exciting to drink.

Rosemary for Remembrance Infusion

Makes 8 cups (64 ounces)   Prep time: 3 minutes

Rosemary is said to improve circulation, soothe a sore throat, and support the mind. Rosemary grows on a small bush, and it is related to mint. It's sturdy, with a strong flavor and aroma. A stem of rosemary looks wonderful in a pitcher of water and adds a delightful taste that doesn't need any muddling to bring it out.

1 large stem of rosemary
2 cups ice
6 cups water

Place the rosemary in a pitcher.

Cover with the ice, then the water.

Leave in the refrigerator for 3 to 12 hours before serving.

Thyme Basil Infusion

The same herbs that offer a bright punch to salad dressings are almost sweet when used as water infusion ingredients. Medicinally, both thyme and basil are used to improve your mood, so you could call this the uplift infusion. Unlike caffeinated drinks, this perky beverage is calming. It can even aid your digestion.

8 to 10 basil leaves
1 stem of thyme leaves
8 cups water

Place the basil leaves and the stem of thyme in a pitcher.

Cover with the water.

Refrigerate for 8 hours before serving.

Lemon Sage Infusion

Sage is an unsung hero of an herb. It's often used in the fall and winter for savory dishes, but it is wonderful year-round. The scientific name for sage comes from the Latin *salvere*, meaning "to save." Sage and lemon create a wonderful infusion that can boost your brain and potentially ward off a cold. Try sage in fruity infusions or alone. Here it gets a wonderful lift from the lemon.

7 to 10 sage leaves
1 lemon, sliced
8 cups water

Place the sage leaves in a pitcher.

Using a long wooden spoon or a muddler, muddle them a little bit for a stronger flavor, if you wish.

Place the lemon slices on top and add the water.

Chill for 3 to 8 hours before serving.

Simply Cinnamon Infusion

Cinnamon-infused water tastes surprising. Is it spicy? Sweet? Invigorating? It seems to be all of those things. While cinnamon pairs nicely with so many ingredients, it is equally fantastic all by itself, and it looks pretty in the pitcher, too. Remember that cinnamon is a warming herb, but as an infusion it is far milder than it would be in a food recipe, so it's nice even on a warm day.

8 cups water
1 cinnamon stick

Simply place the water in a pitcher and add a cinnamon stick.

Refrigerate for 8 to 12 hours before serving.

 You can reuse the cinnamon stick several times.

Herbal Infusions

Marjoram Mint Infusion

Makes 8 cups (64 ounces)   Prep time: 3 minutes

Marjoram is known to relieve stress, insomnia, and menstrual cramps. Infused with mint, this is a delightful herbal beverage that can help with digestion. The amounts here can be adjusted for your personal preference. You can enjoy equal amounts of these herbs, or add more of either one.

10 mint leaves
5 marjoram leaves
8 cups water

Place the leaves and the water into a pitcher.

Refrigerate for 8 to 12 hours.

Mint propagates easily. Take a leaf or two of your favorite variety (mine is chocolate mint) and put it in a glass of water until roots form. Plant it in dirt to have a growing supply.

Lavender
Water Infusion

Lavender is for everyone. Its calming scent can relieve anxiety, depression, and irritability. Lavender is equally tasty in savory or sweet dishes and is wonderful in a pitcher of water. Be sure and get culinary lavender—it will have a better flavor if no pesticides have been used.

2 stems lavender

8 cups water

Place the lavender and water into a pitcher.

Chill for 8 hours before serving.

Lavender often comes in bunches. What you don't infuse can be used in cookies, in scones, or as a beautiful fragrance if you let the flowers dry in a vase.

Herbal Infusions

Lemon Tarragon Infusion

Lemon and tarragon go wonderfully together. The tarragon provides a subtle hint of earthiness that lemon alone doesn't have. Tarragon is said to be good for the eyes and the digestive system. It is especially good for the female reproductive system, but it should not be used during pregnancy.

> 5 tarragon leaves
> 2 lemons, sliced
> 2 cups of ice
> 6 cups of water

Place the tarragon and lemon slices in a pitcher.

Add the ice and then the water.

Infuse in the fridge for 4 to 8 hours before serving.

Parsley Vanilla Infusion

Makes 8 cups (64 ounces)   Prep time: 5 minutes

Here is a combination I bet you never thought of. Bitter parsley rarely gets paired with velvety vanilla. For a refreshing beverage, this infusion brings out a lovely pair of flavors that you will want to taste again and again.

    1 vanilla bean
    4 stems fresh parsley
    8 cups water

Either slice the vanilla bean in half, or muddle a little in a pitcher.

Add the parsley and water.

Refrigerate for 6 to 8 hours before serving.

Dill Infusion

Makes 8 cups (64 ounces)   Prep time: 2 minutes

Dill might make you think of pickles, but this pretty infusion isn't anything like that. It's fun and herbal in a sprightly way. Dill is soothing to the spirit as well as the stomach. It's also great for those who have trouble sleeping, which makes this a simple and practical water infusion.

1 large stem of dill
8 cups water

Place the dill and water into a pitcher.

Refrigerate for 8 hours before serving.

Fruit Infused Water

Basil Mint Infusion

Makes 8 cups (64 ounces)   Prep time: 5 minutes

Basil and mint are cousins in the same family. Paired together, they have a complex and pleasant flavor. Basil is known as a restorative herb that can restore your mental balance. Mint is mildly stimulating and good for digestion. Mint is cooling and basil is warming, so in theory putting them together is neutral, not to mention delicious.

    5 basil leaves
    5 mint leaves
    2 cups ice
    6 cups water

Place the mint and basil in a pitcher.

Muddle for a minute.

Add the ice on top, then the water.

Infuse together for 6 to 8 hours before serving.

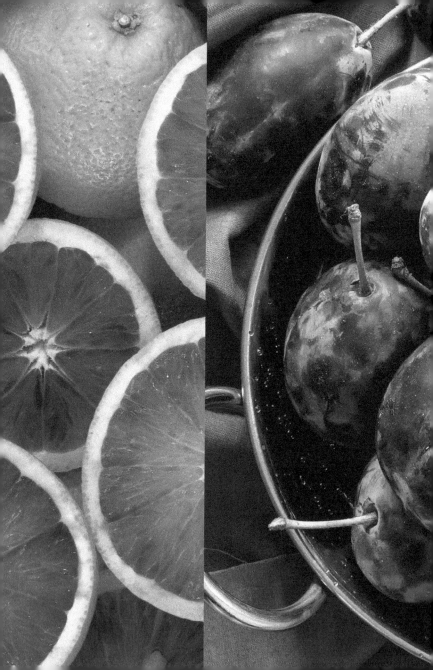

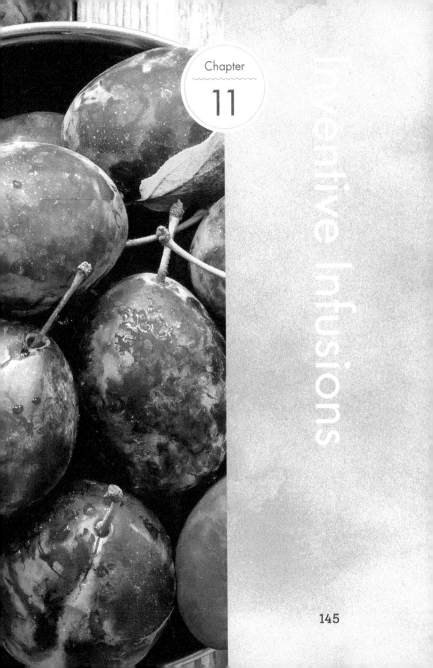

Inventive Infusions

Now it is time to get creative with inventive infusion recipes. The recipes in this book are guides to get you started making your own infusions, designed to spark ideas for new flavor combinations you want to try. Be sure to write down your favorite combinations to remember for later, or flag the ones in this book that you find you like best. Take one of the recipes you like and see what else you might do with it—add an herb or spice, play with a touch of sweetener, or substitute a different type of fruit. What can you do to make that recipe even better?

If you have access to exotic fruits, don't hesitate to try them—they, too, will infuse nicely. Lychees, for example, can be used like grapes, and guava infuses just as well as mango. There are melons grown in Texas that other states never get to taste, and unless you have a Chinatown or an incredible health-food store near you, you might never see the September fruit jujube. If you enjoy exotic fruits, get inventive and see what you come up with. In this chapter you will find recipes made with readily available ingredients that are also inventive in their flavor combinations.

Apple Sage Infusion

Makes 8 cups (64 ounces)   Prep time: 3 minutes

Using fresh sage in anything seems to invoke feelings of fall no matter what time of year it is. This sagely sipper can bring you a gust of that cool fall air even on the hottest day. Apples, a fall fruit, pair beautifully with sage for a unique combination that is both simple and complex. Sage is known for its beneficial effects on menopausal symptoms, but it can be calming for anyone who tends to be anxious.

7 fresh sage leaves
2 apples, cored and sliced
8 cups water

Put the sage leaves in a pitcher and muddle a little.

Add the apple slices and muddle a bit more.

Add the water and chill for 2 to 12 hours before serving.

If you only have dried sage on hand for this recipe, it is not a problem—you can use dried herbs in your infusions in place of fresh herbs. Depending how old the herbs are, however, you might need to adjust the amounts to your taste.

Cocoa Cinnamon Mint Strawberry Infusion

Makes 8 cups (64 ounces)   Prep time: 4 minutes

Zippy cocoa, cinnamon, and mint are a great inventive infusion combo that can definitely perk you up while enjoying a delicious water. Strawberry pairs well with each of these ingredients but will taste best if ripe and sweet. If your fruit isn't as sweet as you like, add a hint of natural sweetener to this recipe or another sweet fruit such as mango or orange.

- 2 cups sliced strawberries
- 3 fresh mint sprigs
- ½ teaspoon cocoa powder
- 1 small cinnamon stick
- 8 cups water

Put the fruit into your pitcher and muddle to release the flavor.

Add the mint, cocoa, and cinnamon stick and pour in the water.

Chill for 2 to 12 hours before serving.

Blueberry Orange Lime Thyme Infusion

Makes 8 cups (64 ounces)   Prep time: 4 minutes

Adding thyme to a fruit infusion yields a unique flavor combination that is terrific as long as you don't overdo the herb. Fresh thyme can bunch up, and it may be tempting to just toss in the whole bunch. Pull the sprigs apart over the sink so that the small needles don't make a mess as you separate your thyme. Instead of overpowering the infusion, using a few sprigs of fresh thyme will mingle well with the blueberry, orange, and lime. This infusion will help soothe the symptoms of a cough or cold.

1 cup fresh blueberries
1 large orange, sliced
1 lime, sliced
3 fresh thyme sprigs
8 cups water

Put the fruits into a pitcher along with the thyme and muddle for 1 minute.

Add the water and chill for 1 to 8 hours before serving.

This infusion pairs particularly well with fish as the main course of your meal, because thyme is often used to flavor seafood.

Rosemary
Pineapple Infusion

Makes 8 cups (64 ounces)   Prep time: 2 minutes

Sweet and bright pineapple gets a lovely kick from
stimulating rosemary leaves. Rosemary has a pungent,
pinelike fragrance that infuses easily and works well with
other potent flavors such as pineapple. One of the many
health benefits of rosemary is that it contains chemicals
that have been shown to boost immune function, improve
digestion, and increase circulation.

2 cups pineapple chunks
2 fresh rosemary sprigs
8 cups water

Muddle the pineapple and rosemary in a pitcher.

Add the water to cover and chill for 1 to 6 hours
before serving.

*Rosemary is also known to make great tea that can be
used as an aspirin alternative for pain. If you let the ingredients for this recipe infuse longer, the beverage will have
more of this special benefit.*

Cocoa Raspberry Tangerine Infusion

Makes 8 cups (64 ounces)   Prep time: 3 minutes

Like most citrus fruits, tangerines are incredibly rich in vitamin C. They also contain a significant amount of flavonoid antioxidants. Raspberries are known for their anti-inflammatory and antioxidant benefits as well as their bright red color. These two ingredients combine with cocoa to create an infusion that has notes of sweetness and bitterness while also being sour and tart. If you cannot find tangerines for this recipe, feel free to use oranges; they will impart a similar flavor and nutrient profile.

2 cups fresh raspberries
1 or 2 tangerines, sliced
½ teaspoon cocoa powder
6 cups ice cubes
2 cups water

Put the fruits and cocoa powder in a pitcher.

Add the ice and water.

Chill for 1 to 6 hours before serving.

Lavender Plum Infusion

Makes 8 cups (64 ounces)   Prep time: 3 minutes

Both plums and lavender are wonderfully fragrant ingredients. Lavender Plum is a simple inventive infusion that might remind you of the slower pace of life in the Victorian era. Don't be surprised if you find yourself looking for a good book and a quiet spot to read as you keep sipping.

1 teaspoon culinary lavender
4 ripe plums, pitted and sliced
8 cups water

Put the lavender and plum slices in a pitcher.

Muddle for 1 minute.

Add the water and chill for 1 to 8 hours before serving.

While reusable shopping bags are environmentally friendly, they are not necessarily the best carriers to use when shopping for fruit. The best option to keep your fruits from bruising may be a wicker shopping basket. They are light and easy to carry, and you can take them on a picnic, too.

Cherry Banana Lime Coconut Infusion

Red, green, and bright white colors give this infusion a colorful party-like appearance in a clear pitcher. The flavors produce an energetic feeling as the sweetness gets sparkly with lime and the notes of tartness mix with heady coconut. This is a flavor-filled combination that might remind you of breakfast on a tropical island or a party on the beach.

1 ripe banana, peeled and sliced
1 cup cherries, pitted
2 limes, sliced
1 cup fresh coconut meat (or ¼ cup dried)
8 cups water

Put the fruits and coconut in a pitcher and muddle for 1 minute.

Add the water and chill for 2 to 8 hours before serving.

Serving water with a straw can help encourage you to drink more. Straws are fun to drink with and are often associated with beverage treats from our past. If you are trying to drink more water, adding a straw just might work for you.

Basil Lemon Fig Infusion

While this might sound almost like a salad dressing, water infused with lemon, basil, and fig is light, sweet, and invigorating. Make sure that you have sweet ripe figs to use and skip the ones that are not soft or are still white inside. It is okay to use figs that have a bit of skin rubbed off and those that have dark spots, indicating that they are very ripe.

Inventive Infusions

    2 cups fresh sliced figs
    1 lemon, sliced
    3 or 4 large fresh basil leaves
    8 cups water

Put the figs in a pitcher with the lemon slices.

Rub the basil leaves between your fingers for a minute to release their flavor and add to the fruits.

Add the water and chill for 1 to 8 hours before serving.

Cranapple Berry Infusion

Makes 8 cups (64 ounces)   Prep time: 6 minutes

Here is one infusion where dried fruit works better than fresh for the cranberries. The berries in this recipe all combine well with the apple to create a light, sweet, and tart infusion. If you love fruity candies like Starburst or SweeTarts, this inventive infusion is one that you will likely enjoy again and again.

½ cup apple-sweetened dried cranberries
1 apple, cored and sliced
1 cup fresh blueberries or blackberries
8 cups water

Put the fruits in a pitcher and muddle for 1 minute.

Add the water and chill for 2 to 12 hours before serving.

To release more flavor from the dried cranberries, you can bunch up the dried fruit with your fingers and then chop it into pieces with a sharp knife.

Tangerine Fig Rosemary Infusion

Sweet figs and tangerines combined with rosemary create an exotic flavor combination that is a mixture of tropical and old world flavors. This infusion tastes like a well-blended mixture of ingredients gathered from around the globe. Any type of citrus would work in this recipe, but tangerine lends itself nicely to the inventive infusions—it is a flavor that doesn't get used often enough.

2 tangerines, sliced
1 cup fresh figs, sliced
1 or 2 fresh rosemary sprigs
8 cups water

Put the tangerines, figs, and rosemary in a pitcher.

Add the water and chill for 2 to 8 hours before serving.

Rosemary bushes can work easily in the landscape of a yard and provide you with both a lovely fragrance and a lifetime supply of fresh rosemary.

Inventive Infusions

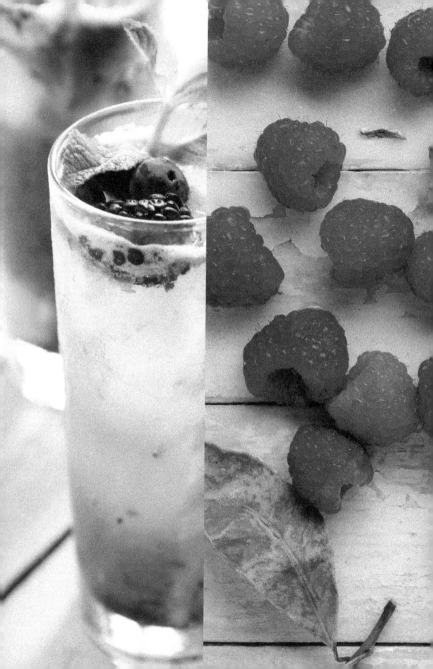

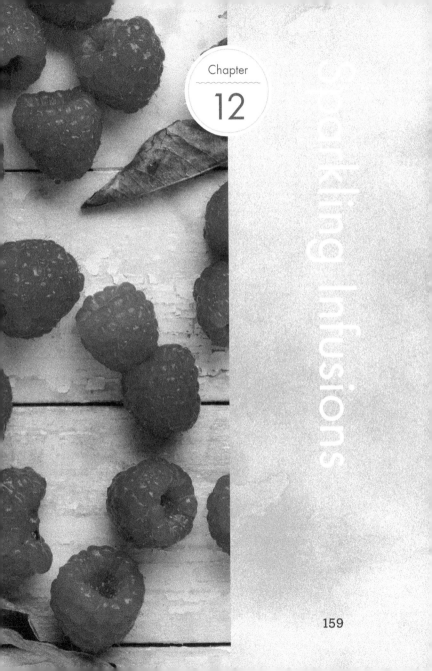

Sparkling Infusions

When CO_2 is added to water, you get a carbonic acid solution, or sparkling water. You may also be familiar with the terms fizzy water, soda water, or seltzer—they are all the same thing. You can purchase a wide variety of sparkling waters with varying degrees of carbonation, or you can make your own fizzy water with a home carbonation product such as the SodaStream. Sparkling water is a fun ingredient that can be enjoyed in moderation as part of a healthy lifestyle. Just be sure you are drinking enough regular water, too!

While the recipes in this chapter are designed specifically to work with sparkling water, most of the previous recipes in this book will work with sparkling water as well. Keep in mind that carbonated water will go flat over time, so if you are not planning to drink all of your sparkling creation within a few hours, you might want to transfer it to a bottle with a tightly sealing lid to keep it from going flat.

Sparkling Grape Pear Infusion

Makes 8 cups (64 ounces)   Prep time: 6 minutes

Infusing sparkling water with fresh grapes and pears yields a delightful beverage that might bring to mind the classic elegance of a 1940s film or a yacht. Pears and grapes just seem to go together so beautifully, and their soft green color is as fresh as their taste.

1 or 2 ripe pears
1 cup green grapes, halved
8 cups sparkling water
Fresh rosemary sprigs, for garnish

Slice the pears and put them in a pitcher.

Muddle for 1 minute, then add the grapes and water.

Chill for 2 hours, then serve in a wine or martini glass with a sprig of rosemary.

If you would like a less bubbly infusion that has added flavor from the fruits, infuse for several hours in 4 cups of still water and then add the 4 cups of sparkling water just before serving.

Sparkling Raspberry Vanilla Infusion

Makes 8 cups (64 ounces)   Prep time: 4 minutes

Infusing raspberries yields a bright flavor that is almost better than eating them fresh. The tiny seeds won't get caught in your teeth, but the wonderful flavor bursts into the sparkling water to combine nicely with vanilla for a flavor that is just as sparkly as the bubbly water itself. You won't miss sodas with any of these sparkling infusions, and this combination is one that is delicious enough for bottling.

1 vanilla bean
2 cups fresh raspberries
8 cups sparkling water

Put the vanilla bean into a pitcher and muddle for 1 minute.

Add the raspberries and muddle for 30 seconds more.

Add the sparkling water and chill for 1 to 3 hours before serving.

Sparkling Persimmon Basil Infusion

Makes 8 cups (64 ounces)   Prep time: 5 minutes

Similar in appearance to little pumpkins with their orange skin and round shape, persimmons are rapidly increasing in popularity and availability. This fruit is said to be an Asian apple, but there are two kinds of persimmon. The fuyu, which has a flat bottom, is crunchy like an apple. The hachiya has a more elongated bottom to give the fruit a teardrop shape and is soft like jelly. Both are sweet and enjoyable when ripe and either will work in infusions.

4 large fresh basil leaves
3 persimmons, sliced
8 cups sparkling water

Put the basil in a pitcher and muddle.

Add the persimmons and muddle again.

Pour in the water and chill for 2 to 6 hours before serving.

If you have to buy persimmons by the bag or the box, freeze any overripe fruit after slicing it in half. You can use the fruit for infusions, or even eat the frozen flesh like a natural sorbet.

Sparkling Pomegranate Mint Infusion

Pomegranate is turning up in juices, desserts, salads, and savory dishes with increasing regularity. This fruit is fun to eat, and it has a sweet but tart flavor that lends itself perfectly to infused water—it has a lovely color, too. Trader Joe's carries containers of pomegranate already peeled and ready to eat.

5 to 9 fresh mint leaves
½ cup pomegranate (or 1 whole fruit, peeled and
    seeds separated)
8 cups sparkling water

Put the mint into your pitcher and muddle for 1 minute.

Add the pomegranate and muddle for 1 minute more.

Add the sparkling water and chill for 1 to 4 hours before serving.

Fresh pomegranate is rich in antioxidants, which have added benefits for the skin such as sun protection, supporting cell regeneration, and increasing moisture.

Sparkling Pineapple Lemonade Infusion

Makes 8 cups (64 ounces)   Prep time: 3 minutes

Sparkling lemonade gets a zippy twist in this recipe from the addition of fresh pineapple. Since pineapple is very sweet, you might not need the added sweetener. Because this is an infusion and not juice, or fruit blended with water, the taste is light enough that you can enjoy more of it than you would with regular lemonade.

2 cups fresh pineapple chunks
3 lemons, sliced
Stevia, honey, or agave (optional)
8 cups sparkling water

Put the fruit in a pitcher and muddle for 1 minute.

Add the sweetener (if using) and the water.

Chill for 1 to 3 hours before serving.

Frozen pineapple chunks can be used in place of fresh if necessary, but dried pineapple will not impart the same zippy flavor.

Sparkling Cocoa Cherry Grape Infusion

This recipe might remind you of a cola, but it's much healthier. Feel free to add a bit of sweetener for an extra punch, but with both cherries and grapes to balance out the bitterness of the cocoa, it's already refreshing and full of flavor.

- ½ cup cherries, pitted and halved
- ½ cup grapes, halved
- 1 tablespoon cocoa nibs
- 8 cups sparkling water

Place the fruits and cocoa in a pitcher.

You may wish to muddle them for added flavor.

Add the sparkling water and chill for 3 to 8 hours before serving.

Sparkling Infusions

 If you don't have nibs, use cocoa powder instead.

Sparkling Peach Cranberry Lime Infusion

Here is a fruity combination that is fit for a feast. If you use frozen cranberries or peaches instead of fresh ones, you will need to let them defrost before you muddle them.

- ½ cup cranberries
- 1 cup peach chunks or slices
- 1 lime, sliced
- 8 cups sparkling water

Place the cranberries and peaches in a pitcher.

Muddle the fruit to release the flavors into your water.

Add the lime and water.

Chill for 1 to 8 hours before serving.

Alternatively to muddling the berries, you could pierce each with a sharp knife.

Fruit Infused Water

Sparkling Mango Coconut Infusion

This tropical infusion is best when you use sweet, ripe fruit. If you are using a whole fresh coconut, you can include the milk from the fruit as well.

½ cup coconut chunks
1 cup mango, cut into chunks or cubes
8 cups sparkling water

Place the fruit into a pitcher.

You may muddle a little if you wish. With very ripe fruit, it is not necessary.

Refrigerate for 1 to 8 hours before serving.

Set off this sparkling infusion with the bright color of mint or strawberry as a garnish.

Sparkling Infusions

Sparkling Strawberry Pineapple Infusion

Makes 8 cups (64 ounces)   Prep time: 4 minutes

This sweet and fruity infusion is like a party in your mouth. Use the most flavorful strawberries of the bunch. You'll recognize them by their rich red appearance and the absence of white spots. Pick the pineapple chunks that have a dark yellow appearance.

- 1 cup strawberries, halved or sliced with stems and leaves removed
- 1 cup pineapple chunks
- 8 cups sparkling water

Put the fruit in a pitcher.

Muddle the fruit to release the flavors more fully.

Add the water and chill for 1 to 6 hours before serving.

Leave half of the berries unmuddled for their pretty appearance, or add a few extra berry slices before serving.

Fruit Infused Water

Sparkling Apple Grape Blueberry Infusion

Makes 8 cups (64 ounces)   Prep time: 7 minutes

Use your favorite apples and your favorite grapes in this recipe. Both green and red grapes work well, and they pair beautifully with blueberries. This recipe works for any season. It's high in antioxidants and sweet in flavor. When fresh blueberries aren't available, you can use frozen ones.

1 apple, sliced
½ cup blueberries
½ cup grapes
8 cups sparkling water

Place the apple slices in a pitcher and muddle.

Add the blueberries and grapes and muddle more.

Add the sparkling water and chill for 1 to 8 hours before serving.

You might want to make a large amount overnight by using enough still water to cover the fruits, then add sparkling water just before serving to equal 8 cups.

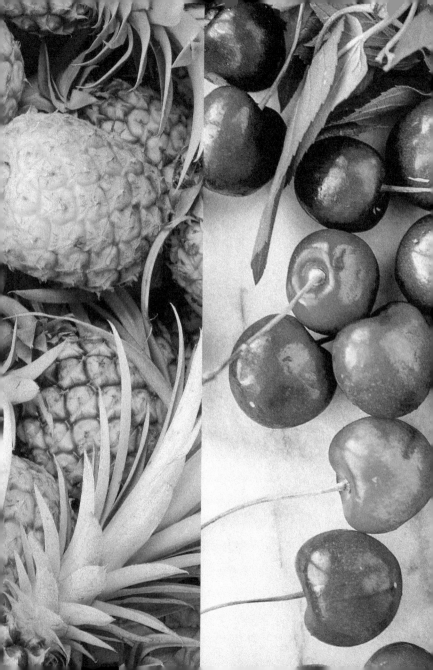

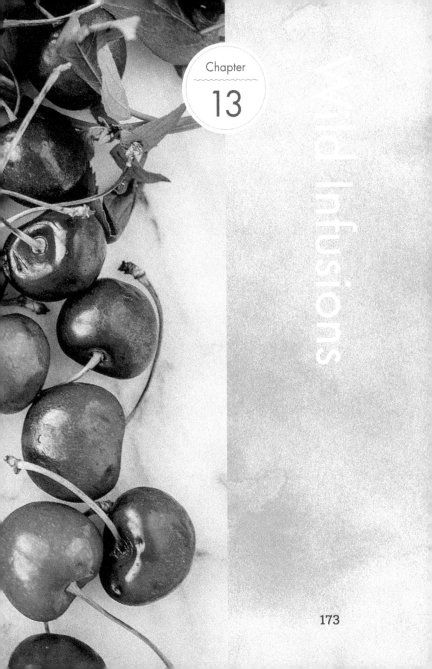

Wild Infusions

Get ready to go wild with flavors in your fruit infusions. Eating should be fun, and when you make water infusions that you love to drink, you will not only enjoy the health benefits of drinking more water and fresh nutrients, you will also brighten up your day. Here are some examples of really fun fruity inventions.

Some of these recipes are inspired by candy or other treats, but do not expect your water infusions to be a carbon copy of those candy flavors—they were just the inspiration.

After you've experimented with these recipes, you can modify them and come up with your own favorites. Be willing to experiment to see what happens when you mix things. If you don't like what you made, chalk it up to being a scientist on the road to genius. The more flavor combinations you try, the more you will learn what works for you.

Fruit Juice Infusion

Makes 8 cups (64 ounces)   Prep time: 7 minutes

Juicy Fruit gum has been around since the 1890s. The company has never revealed whether the gum's flavor is a fruity combination, like this recipe, or a single flavor of jackfruit that is popular in countries such as Indonesia. New flavors of Juicy Fruit have been introduced, but the original has survived all this time. Here's your own secret fruity water infusion blend. See if sipping it with a straw makes you think of the tropics.

- 1 banana, peeled and sliced
- 1 cup pineapple chunks
- 1 ripe peach, pitted and cut into chunks
- 8 cups water

Place the cut fruit into a pitcher.

Muddle if you wish, for added flavor.

Add the water.

Refrigerate for 2 to 8 hours before serving.

Banana Split Infusion

This is an infusion, not a confection. The flavors are gentle reminders of a banana split. It has all the delicate tones of those great flavors without any of the calories.

    1 banana, peeled and sliced
    ¼ cup pitted sliced cherries
    1 teaspoon cocoa nibs
    ½ teaspoon vanilla extract
    Stevia or other sweetener to taste (optional)
    8 cups water

Place the fruits into a pitcher.

Muddle the fruits.

Add the other ingredients.

Refrigerate for 3 to 6 hours before serving.

Try different sweeteners and amounts of fruit to get the flavor closer to what you enjoy about a banana split.

Wild Infusions

Honey & Oats Infusion

Makes 8 cups (64 ounces)   Prep time: 5 minutes

Breakfast cereals make mornings fun, but who says you have to limit them to breakfast? Creating water infusions with your favorite flavors is a healthy way to enjoy the sometimes silly things we only allow ourselves when we first get up. This water infusion, inspired by Honey Nut Cheerios and Honey Bunches of Oats, brings out your inner child. Just don't start wearing a bee costume.

1 cup rolled oats
½ cup raw honey (use brown rice syrup for a
    vegan option)
1 teaspoon vanilla extract or 1 vanilla bean cut in half
    (optional)
8 cups water

Place all of the ingredients in a pitcher.

Refrigerate for 3 to 6 hours before serving.

There are many varieties of raw honey. All have great health benefits, and each has a unique flavor. Experiment to find one you like best. Often, the darker the honey, the richer the flavor.

Caribbean Pops Infusion

Makes 8 cups (64 ounces)   Prep time: 3 minutes

Picture yourself on a balmy island as you sip this tropical blend. With this recipe you can enjoy all the island flavor without the sugar that normally goes with it.

    ½ cup strawberries, sliced
    1 mango, pitted and sliced
    ½ cup pineapple, cubed
    ½ cup fresh coconut, cubed
    8 cups water

Place the fruits in a pitcher.

Muddle if desired.

Add the coconut.

Add the water.

Refrigerate for 3 to 8 hours before serving.

Splendid Almond Infusion

Makes 8 cups (64 ounces)   Prep time: 5 minutes

You may want to use blanched almonds for this Almond Joy–inspired recipe, as the almond skins will come off and float after being soaked. Removing the skins will remove bitterness from your beverage and give you more of the almond flavor. For extra almond taste, chop the almonds before infusing them.

1 cup almonds
¼ cup cocoa nibs
½ cup fresh coconut
8 cups water

Place all of the ingredients into a pitcher.

Refrigerate for 6 to 12 hours before serving.

You can muddle the ingredients for additional flavor before adding the water. For even stronger flavor, you can pulse the ingredients in a food processor, infuse, and strain before serving.

Fruit Burst Infusion

Starburst comes in so many great flavors. Nothing can match unwrapping one of those individual squares and getting to savor its chewiness, but this water infusion has a great wild fruit flavor that won't stick to your teeth or spoil your dinner.

½ cup strawberries
½ cup grapes
½ cup cherries
1 vanilla bean, sliced in half
8 cups water

Place the fruits and vanilla in a pitcher.

Muddle a little.

Cover with the water.

Chill for 2 to 12 hours before serving.

Rainbow Infusion

Here you can "taste the rainbow" of sweet, fruity flavors with a hint of soft clouds thrown in. For a soft pink flavor, add a handful of fresh cherries to the mix.

> 1–2 oranges, sliced
> ½ cup grapes, sliced
> 1 vanilla bean sliced in half
> 8 cups water

Place all of the ingredients into a pitcher.

Refrigerate for 3 to 12 hours before serving.

Fruit Infused Water

If you are serving a Rainbow Infusion at a party, you can add one drop of natural food coloring to give it a strong color. Use a different color for each pitcher that you make.

Lemon Pie Infusion

Makes 8 cups (64 ounces)   Prep time: 3 minutes

A hint of vanilla and sweetener in this lemon water infusion makes it more like a lemon pie. It's light and sparkly on its own and equally fun mixed with sparkling water instead of flat.

    3 lemons, sliced
    1 vanilla bean, cut in half
    1 to 2 teaspoons stevia
    8 cups water

Place half the lemon slices into a pitcher.

Muddle the lemon.

Add the rest of the lemon along with the other ingredients.

Chill for 3 to 12 hours before serving.

You can reuse these ingredients to make additional pitchers. If you muddle it again and most of the lemon slices get broken down the second or third time, that's fine. Just fill it with water and chill.

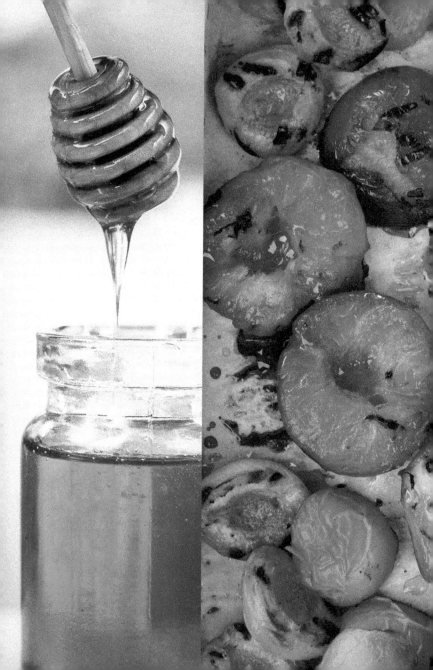

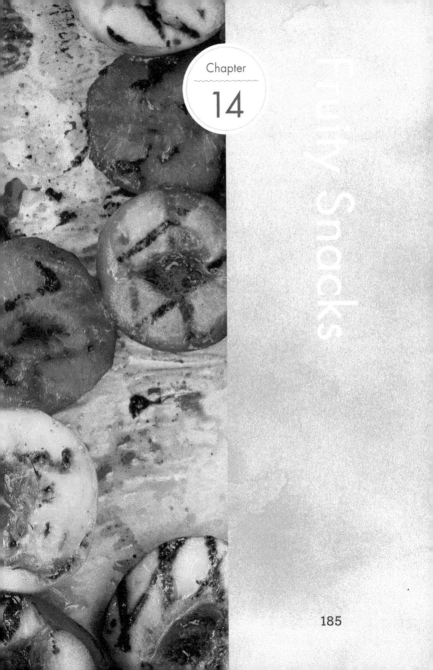

Fruity Snacks

You might have so much fun purchasing fruits and herbs for water infusions that you have ripe fruits left over. This chapter is full of fun ways to enjoy your produce and make sure it gets used.

Of course you can always eat fresh fruit on its own. Berries are best when they're recently picked, as they lose their sweetness the longer they sit. Over-ripe fruits can still be wonderful in water infusion, but if you have purchased more than you can use (maybe you got an incredible deal at a roadside stand, or went to a pick-your-own farm) the freezer is a good option, too.

These recipes are guidelines that you can use to create a variety of delicious, healthy snacks. Experiment with your favorite combinations and use what you have on hand. You can add your favorite herbs and spices as well. Some people like a bit of salt in their fruit snacks to bring out the sweetness or create an opposition of flavors. Or you might find you want to add mint to everything. Adjust and make yourself happy, because fruit is always supposed to be a treat.

Fruit Pockets

Makes 1 pocket   Prep time: 10 minutes

These fun fruit pockets can be a quick snack for one person, or you can make enough for a party and serve them with your favorite ice cream.

  1 rice wrap (may be called spring roll skin)
  ¼ to ½ cup berries, washed and stems removed
  ¼ to ½ cup sweet fruit (kiwi, pineapple, mango, etc.)
  ½ small lemon
  Honey to drizzle
  1 large basil leaf (optional)

Heat an inch of water in a large skillet until tiny bubbles begin to form.

Add your rice wrap for a minute to soften, and remove carefully so as not to tear it.

Place on a plate or cutting board.

Add the fruits to the center of the wrap.

Squeeze a little lemon onto the fruit and drizzle with honey.

If using a basil leaf, cut into fine strips and sprinkle on top.

Fold the wrap as you would a burrito, pulling in all sides.

For an extra treat, drizzle chocolate sauce over the top of the pocket before serving.

Juice Pops

Juice pops are a fun treat and so simple to make. Here I've used grape juice for its flavor and rich color, but of course you could use any juice you like. Unlike most store-bought pops, this version has no added sugar. You might want to make several trays of these and then keep them in a freezer bag.

> 1½ cups pure purple grape juice with nothing added
> 10 berries or small fruit chunks
> Toothpicks

Using an ice cube tray, pour the grape juice into each cup until three-quarters full.

Add one berry or small fruit chunk to each.

Stick the toothpick into the fruit in the center of each cup.

Freeze until solid.

You can use wooden tongue-depressor sticks instead of toothpicks to have a larger surface to hold onto.

Fresh Frozen Persimmon Cups

Makes 8 servings   Prep time: 2 minutes

My grandmother served a lot of "fresh frozen" fruits and vegetables. She said it was better than fresh, because she loved the convenience of being able to purchase her favorite items year-round. Here we are using the freezer to make fun frozen treats out of fresh produce. In this simple persimmon recipe, the freezer magically transforms the ripe fruit into an instant sorbet. You don't need a blender or anything special. Just slice, freeze, and enjoy.

4 persimmons—very ripe

Cut each persimmon in half.

Place in the freezer overnight.

Using the peel as a cup, eat the frozen fruit with a spoon.

Mint and Honey
Fruit Salad

Makes 4 cups (32 ounces)   Prep time: 10 minutes

Fruit salads make fun snacks or desserts. They are light, sweet, refreshing, and wonderfully healthy. Feel free to use the fruits you have on hand—this is just a guide. You could make a salad with different types of melon, or do a tropical salad with all tropical fruits. This is a mix of items I had on hand one day, and it worked well.

- 1 cup blueberries
- 1 cup apple, cored and cut into chunks
- 1 cup pineapple, cut into chunks
- 1 cup pear, cored and cut into chunks
- 2 limes
- 2 tablespoons honey
- 5 mint leaves, chopped

Place all of the fruit into a large bowl.

Squeeze the juice of the limes over the fruit.

Drizzle the honey over the fruit.

Add the chopped mint.

Mix well.

1 Hour Apple Chips

Makes 9 servings   Prep time: 5 minutes

Apples are fun snacks when they're freshly picked or when they're dehydrated. You don't need any fancy equipment to get the same great apple chips you might find in a store. When you make them yourself, you can add anything you like. If you don't love cinnamon, for example, leave it out, or try nutmeg instead. Be sure to check your apple chips toward the end of cooking to make sure they do not brown too much. Every oven is different and yours might run hot or cool, so adjust cooking times accordingly.

3 large apples, cored and sliced thin
1 teaspoon cinnamon

Preheat oven to 225°F.

Place the apple slices in a bowl and sprinkle with cinnamon.

Mix to get cinnamon on all of the slices.

Place the apples on baking sheets lined with parchment paper in a single layer.

Bake for 1 hour.

Grilled Fruit

Makes 8 servings   Prep time: 2 minutes

Grilled fruit is one of those special summertime treats. Pick your fruit, or grill several on skewers. This is one of those easy-to-do recipes that often gets overlooked, as the grill gets reserved for burgers or hot dogs. Grilling fruits caramelizes the sugars and creates a very distinct sweetness. It's comforting and satisfying, and it doesn't heat up the kitchen.

4 peaches, pitted and sliced in half
or
8 watermelon wedges

Simply place the fruit on the grill.

Grill for 2 to 3 minutes on each side.

Fillo Parfait Cups

Makes 12 cups   Prep time: 15 minutes

You can find mini fillo pastry cups in the freezer that are already baked and ready to go. They defrost quickly, and I've even made this recipe without waiting for them to be fully defrosted before I begin filling the cups. I just let them sit out for a few extra minutes, and they were wonderful. Here again is a great fruit snack that makes an elegant dessert.

1 package of mini fillo dough shells
2 cups yogurt (use your favorite plain or fruit-free variety)
2 cups fruit (sliced or chopped)

Defrost your fillo dough shells for 5 minutes by simply removing them from the freezer and leaving them on the counter. It helps to remove them from the packaging.

Fill each cup half full with yogurt.

Place the fruits on top of the yogurt.

If you are serving these for a gathering, garnish with a sprinkle of mint, basil, or dark chocolate.

Fruit Sushi Rolls

These fun fruit creations are a little more work than others, but they're worth it because they're so fun to eat. You can make them with melons instead of papaya, and of course fill them with any fruits that will slice into matchstick pieces. You can add a chocolate dipping sauce if you want to.

1 papaya, ripe but not overripe
1 green apple, cored and sliced into matchstick pieces

Cut away the peel of the papaya. Using a peeler, cut 8 to 12 strips of fruit.

Roll up a few of the apple sticks into each papaya strip and stand on end to serve.

Continue until you have used up all of the apple.

Fruity Snacks

Nutty Bites

Makes 4 servings   Prep time: 6–8 minutes

Nutty and sweet foods go well together. Kids love these treats as much as adults. Get creative and come up with your own variations. The raspberries add a splash of color that makes serving these together more cheery.

> 2 ripe bananas, peeled and sliced into rounds
> ½ cup nut butter (almond, cashew, etc.)
> ½ cup raspberries

Take one banana round and spread a thin amount of nut butter on one side.

Top with another banana slice.

Take a raspberry and fill the hollow center with a dab of nut butter.

Serve with toothpicks.

You can load each bite onto a toothpick before serving and even put one filled raspberry on top of each banana sandwich.

Fruit Sushi Sticks

Makes 4 servings   Prep time: 10 minutes

One thing that makes sushi enjoyable is the bite-sized combinations of flavor. You can do endless variations on fruit sushi, too. Because fruits are often slippery and do not stay together well, I've added the toothpicks to make this recipe easier to eat. Experiment with using different herbs such as thyme instead of mint, or other citrus fruits in place of the orange, and of course whatever fruits you have on hand.

½ cup ripe blackberries
½ melon or papaya, cut into small chunky rectangles
   or cubes
2 large mint leaves, sliced
1 orange

Place one blackberry on top of each rectangle of melon (or papaya).

Sprinkle a few think slices of mint on top.

Place a toothpick through the fruits to hold them together.

Squeeze the juice from the orange on top.

You can dip each of these in chocolate sauce before eating.

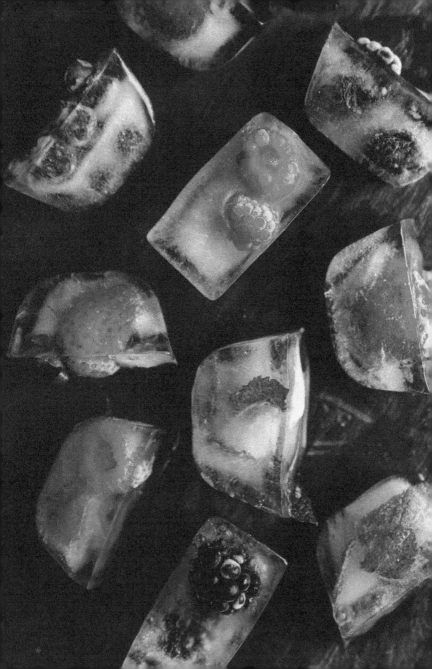

Acknowledgments

It takes a village to raise a book—even a relatively small book of recipes. Thank you to Brian Hurley and the wonderful Callisto Media team. Judith Bruce for a great place to live. My students and fans—you always inspire me to keep creating. And a huge thank-you to my parents, who always encouraged me to enjoy the kitchen, have an appreciation for healthy foods, and were my first teachers in picking the best produce. Your love is in everything I make.

Resources

Books

Wood, Rebecca. *The New Whole Foods Encyclopedia: A Comprehensive Resource for Healthy Eating.* Penguin Books, 1999.

Articles and Websites

Answers.com. "Cucumbers, Melons and Other Cucurbits." Accessed July 3, 2014. http://www.encyclopedia.com /doc/1G2-3403400167.html

Davis, Jeanie Lerche. "Cranberries: Year-Round Superfood." WebMD. Accessed July 3, 2014. http://www .webmd.com/food-recipes/features/cranberries-year -round-superfood

Guilford, Carolyn. "The Skinny on Stevia." *Savannah Morning News.* April 15, 2014. ProQuest. Accessed June 10, 2014.

HealthAlternatives.com. "Vitamin Chart." Accessed July 3, 2014. http://www.health-alternatives.com/vitamins -nutrition-chart.html

Hendrick, Bill. "Cocoa Rich in Health Benefits." WebMD. Accessed July 3, 2014. http://www.webmd.com/diabetes/news/20110323/cocoa-rich-in-health-benefits

Huff, James, Michael F. Jacobson, and Devra Lee Davis. "Aspartame Bioassay Findings Portend Human Cancer Hazards." *International Journal of Occupational and Environmental Health* 13, no. 4 (Oct.–Dec. 2007): 446–48.

Institute of Medicine. "Dietary Reference Intakes: Water, Potassium, Sodium, Chloride, and Sulfate." Accessed July 3, 2014. http://www.iom.edu/Reports/2004/Dietary-Reference-Intakes-Water-Potassium-Sodium-Chloride-and-Sulfate.aspx

Kadlovski, Shannon. "Coco-Nutty: Are Coconuts Good for You?" Huffpost Living. Accessed July 3, 2014. http://www.huffingtonpost.ca/shannon-kadlovski/coconut-recipes_b_2573556.html

MacPherson, Kitta. "Sugar Can Be Addictive, Princeton Scientist Says." Princeton University News. Accessed July 3, 2014. http://www.princeton.edu/main/news/archive/S22/88/56G31/index.xml?section=topstories

Margen, Sheldon and Dale A. Ogar. "Fresh or Dried, Figs Are Nearly Perfect Fruit." *LA Times.* Accessed July 3, 2014. http://articles.latimes.com/1999/jan/11/health/he-62368

Mayo Clinic. "Organic Food: Is It More Nutritious?" Accessed July 3, 2014. http://www.mayoclinic.org /healthy-living/nutrition-and-healthy-eating/in-depth /organic-food/art-20043880?pg=2

Med-Health.net. "Coconut Meat." Accessed July 3, 2014. http://www.med-health.net/Coconut-Meat.html

MedlinePlus. "Antioxidants." Accessed July 3, 2014. http://www.nlm.nih.gov/medlineplus/antioxidants.html

National Cancer Institute. "Antioxidants and Cancer Prevention." Accessed July 3, 2014. http://www.cancer .gov/cancertopics/factsheet/prevention/antioxidants

NutritionFacts.org. "Fresh Fruit Versus Frozen—Which Is Better?" Accessed July 3, 2014. http://nutritionfacts.org /questions/fresh-fruit-versus-frozen-fruit-which-is -better/?

Obenschain, Chris. "Wondrous Ways that Water Can Improve Your Health." *U.S. News.* Accessed July 3, 2014. http://health.usnews.com/health-news/articles /2012/07/17/wondrous-ways-that-water-can-improve -your-health

Organic Facts. "Health Benefits of Organic Food." Accessed July 3, 2014. http://www.organicfacts.net /organic-food/health-benefits-of-organic-food.html

Schomer, Stephanie. "The Sweet Lowdown: Exposing the Unhealthy Truth About Sugar." Oprah.com. Accessed July 3, 2014. http://www.oprah.com/health/Health-Risks-of-Sugar-Robert-Lustig-Interview_1

Shapley, Dan. "The New Dirty Dozen: 12 Foods to Eat Organic." *Good Housekeeping*. Accessed July 3, 2014. http://www.goodhousekeeping.com/recipes/healthy/dirty-dozen-foods#slide-2

Shaw, Gina. "What Are the Best Sources of Drinking Water?" WebMD. Accessed July 3, 2014. http://www.webmd.com/diet/features/best-sources-drinking-water

WebMD. "Vanilla." Accessed July 3, 2014. http://www.webmd.com/vitamins-supplements/ingredientmono-206-VANILLA.aspx?activeIngredientId=206&activeIngredientName=VANILLA

Weil, Andrew. "Organic Foods Have More Antioxidants, Minerals." Weekly Bulletin. Accessed July 3, 2014. http://www.drweil.com/drw/u/WBL02077/Organic-Foods-Have-More-Antioxidants-Minerals.html

William Mitchell College of Law, Public Health Law Center. "Sickly Sweet: Why the Focus on Sugary Drinks." Accessed July 3, 2014. http://publichealthlawcenter.org/sites/default/files/resources/phlc-fs-Healthy%20Bevs_Sickly%20Sweet%20June%202013.pdf

Resources for Equipment and Ingredients

Farmers' Market

Getting fresh produce from your local farmers' market or health food shop is a great way to go. Search for a farmers' market at:

http://www.localharvest.org

Local Coops

Local Coops are also terrific places to get food, and most have membership for added discounts. Often you do not need to be a member to shop there:

http://www.coopdirectory.org/directory.htm

Water Infusion Pitchers

Water infusion pitchers are a great investment—they will make infusions and other beverages easier to make and to clean up. They will save you time and frustration. In some cases these types of pitchers help get the most from your fruit, too.

Primula Flavor It Pitcher—3 in 1 Beverage System

http://primulaproducts.com/teaware/primula-flavor-it-3-in-1-beverage-system.html

http://www1.macys.com/shop/product/primula-flavor-it
-3-in-1-beverage-system?ID=752956

Prodyne Iced Fruit Infusion Pitcher

http://www.bedbathandbeyond.com/1/1/46149-prodyne
-iced-fruit-infusion-pitcher.html

http://www.amazon.com/Prodyne-Infusion-93-Ounce
-Natural-Pitcher/dp/B0023UL86A/ref=sr_1_1?s=home
-garden&ie=UTF8&qid=1403469053&sr=1-1&keywords
=prodyne+fruit+infusion+93-ounce+natural+fruit
+flavor+pitcher

Target Fruit Infusion Pitcher

http://www.target.com/p/fruit-infusion-pitcher
/-/A-11209652#prodSlot=medium_1_1&term=fruit
+infusion+water+pitcher

Zing Anything

http://www.zinganything.com

http://www.luckyvitamin.com/p-339901-zing-anything
-aqua-zinger-flavored-water-maker-green-20-oz

The Dirty Dozen and the Clean Fifteen

A nonprofit and environmental watchdog organization called Environmental Working Group (EWG) looks at data supplied by the US Department of Agriculture (USDA) and the Food and Drug Administration (FDA) about pesticide residues and compiles a list each year of the best and worst pesticide loads found in commercial crops. You can refer to the Dirty Dozen list to know which fruits and vegetables you should always buy organic. The Clean Fifteen list lets you know which produce is considered safe enough when grown conventionally to allow you to skip the organics. This does not mean that the Clean Fifteen produce is pesticide-free, though, so wash these fruits and vegetables thoroughly. These lists change every year, so make sure you look up the most recent before you fill your shopping cart. You'll find the most recent lists as well as a guide to pesticides in produce at EWG.org/FoodNews.

2015	
DIRTY DOZEN	**CLEAN FIFTEEN**
Apples	Asparagus
Celery	Avocados
Cherry tomatoes	Cabbage
Cucumbers	Cantaloupe
Grapes	Cauliflower
Nectarines	Eggplant
Peaches	Grapefruit
Potatoes	Kiwis
Snap peas	Mangoes
Spinach	Onions
Strawberries	Papayas
Sweet bell peppers	Pineapples
	Sweet corn
In addition to the Dirty Dozen, the EWG added two foods contaminated with highly toxic organophosphate insecticides:	Sweet peas (frozen)
	Sweet potatoes
Hot peppers	
Kale/Collard greens	

Measurement Conversions

Weight Equivalents

US STANDARD	METRIC (APPROXIMATE)
½ ounce	15 g
1 ounce	30 g
2 ounces	60 g
4 ounces	115 g
8 ounces	225 g
12 ounces	340 g
16 ounces or 1 pound	455 g

Volume Equivalents (Liquid)

US STANDARD	US STANDARD (OUNCES)	METRIC (APPROXIMATE)
2 tablespoons	1 fl. oz.	30 mL
¼ cup	2 fl. oz.	60 mL
½ cup	4 fl. oz.	120 mL
1 cup	8 fl. oz.	240 mL
1½ cups	12 fl. oz.	355 mL
2 cups or 1 pint	16 fl. oz.	475 mL
4 cups or 1 quart	32 fl. oz.	1 L
1 gallon	128 fl. oz.	4 L

Volume Equivalents (Dry)

US STANDARD	METRIC (APPROXIMATE)
⅛ teaspoon	.5 mL
¼ teaspoon	1 mL
½ teaspoon	2 mL
¾ teaspoon	4 mL
1 teaspoon	5 mL
1 tablespoon	15 mL
¼ cup	59 mL
⅓ cup	79 mL
½ cup	118 mL
⅔ cup	156 mL
¾ cup	177 mL
1 cup	235 mL
2 cups or 1 pint	475 mL
3 cups	700 mL
4 cups or 1 quart	1 L
½ gallon	2 L
1 gallon	4 L

Recipe Index

Ingredient Index